KETO DIET COOKBOOK FOR WOMEN AFTER 50

THE ULTIMATE GUIDE WITH 151 TASTY LOW-CARB RECIPES TO LOSE WEIGHT FAST. A SIMPLE AND EFFECTIVE METHOD TO FACE MENOPAUSE, RESET METABOLISM AND BOOST YOUR HEALTH

ELIZABETH MEYLIGHT

Table of Contents

Introduction

Growing old is part of life, but one can retain an active and healthy lifestyle long into your later years.

The aging process affects the body in many ways. As we age, our bodies undergo a variety of changes. Our hair begins to gray; our skin loses its elasticity, and wrinkles develop. Muscle loss, reduced stomach acids, and thinning skin are all a part of the aging process. Most of the changes will make you more susceptible to weight gain while also causing nutrient deficiencies. For example, reduced acids in your stomach can affect how nutrients are being absorbed, such as Iron, Vitamin B12, calcium, and magnesium.

Compounding these issues is that as we age, our bodies require less fuel, and we need to decrease the number of calories we eat in a day. This makes it challenging to make sure we get the nutrients needed while eating fewer calories. It's a bit of a nutritional dilemma.

Lucky for us, there are several steps you can do to prevent deficiencies and other age-related changes. As an example, consuming food that is rich in nutrients and ingesting the right supplements can aid in keeping you healthy as you age. Following a Keto-diet is one great way of staying healthy as you continue to age.

The choices we make regarding our food on a day-to-day basis and over our lifetime will always matter more than ever. It may occur to you that since the Keto diet does not allow processed foods and carbohydrates that it is a highly restrictive diet. The Keto diet is not restrictive, as far as diet plans go. As long as you stay in the allowed food groups, you will be given free rein to decide what you want to eat. You will not be experience boredom since choices of food because there are so many choices available. Here in this book, we will be listing down all the foods you can and can't eat.

Everyone knows that watching what you eat and staying active is vital to a healthy lifestyle. However, as we age, things just aren't that simple. Our nutritional needs evolve. Many women find themselves suffering from physical disorders that can make it difficult to swallow, digest foods properly, or find themselves with a significantly reduced appetite.

Your diet is linked to your immune function; it influences mental health and is critical in maintaining healthy bones and sharp eyes. That means women over 50 should make eating a healthy diet suitable to their specific needs.

The ketogenic diet is not just a diet —it is a healthy, weight-reducing way of life. This diet can help you to not only lose weight but control blood pressure, increase mental focus, boost energy, and improve overall health. Keto success is achieved by following low-carbohydrate principles.

Developing and implementing a Keto-friendly diet plan will help to ensure that you are eating nutrient-rich foods while eliminating calorie-dense foods that hold no nutritional value.

Because of its focus on eating nutrient-dense foods, the Keto-diet is perfect for women over 50. With some tweaking and a few minor adjustments to reduce caloric intake and extra nutritional needs, this diet can be tailored to meet everyone's individual needs.
Read this guide for more on how to approach the Keto diet after 50.

Chapter 1: Basic Principles of Keto Diet

The thing about the foods on the Keto Diet is that they deliver a ton of great nutrition and are packed with nutrients. If you have heard of superfoods, well, the Keto Diet is all about leveraging the food you eat for maximum benefit. But even though seniors need fewer calories than their younger counterparts, they do need the same amount of nutrients, and that is a place where the Keto Diet is of great assistance.

The reality is that women aged 50 and older will not have an easy time living on junk food the way they could when they were younger. The body does not snap back the way it once did, and that is why seniors need to be more conscious about the food they are putting in their bodies. The food needs to support their health and fight disease. It is where the quality of life is found and where they can enjoy the years they worked to. Why not spend them in enjoyment instead of being in pain and torment because your diet compromises your ability to enjoy yourself? That is why the Ketogenic diet was built to provide a better and much healthier lifestyle they could ever ask.

When going with the Keto Diet, what ends up happening is that Ketosis helps older people get the nutrition they need to make the most of their senior years instead of suffering through them and lamenting how they can't do what they did when they were younger. It is not how anyone intended to live in their retirement.

Achieving Ketosis is not as simple as it may sound. Ketosis is achieved when your body starts using ketones instead of glucose as fuel. The liver breaks down excess fat stored in the body to make ketones. This metabolic condition occurs when carbohydrates in the body are low and are replaced by fats instead. As an older woman on a keto diet, you will realize that your appetite tends to be suppressed due to the foods you eat, and this feeling of fullness causes you to eat less, causing you to lose weight when fats are broken down.

Ketosis not only benefits your body by making you shed some weight, but it also reduces the risk of diseases such as diabetes and blood pressure. Your question now is how to achieve this state of Ketosis to enjoy all its benefits fully. Follow the following simple steps to get into Ketosis quickly:

Limit Your Carbohydrate Intake

A keto diet is simply a low carbohydrate diet where you increase your fat intake, moderate protein intake, and lower carbohydrate intake. As a woman at 50 years of age or older, you should look forward to reducing your daily carbohydrate intake by consuming foods and drinks that are keto-friendly. For you to achieve Ketosis, your daily carbohydrate intake should fall to as low as between 5-10% of your entire diet.

Upon lowering your carbohydrate intake, your body will be left with minimal carbohydrates to convert into glucose, and it will have no other option than to break down the excess fats to produce ketones through Ketosis.

Increase Your Intake of Healthy Fats

After lowering your carbohydrate intake, your body may become weak if the necessary alternative measures are not taken. That's why you need to ensure you consume enough food, eating enough healthy fat to substitute for the missing carbohydrates.

Consuming the right fatty foods helps regulate your appetite by giving you a feeling of fullness. With a controlled appetite, now and then, you will not need to eat. It gives your body a favorable environment to break down excess fats, making you shed some weight.

Moderate Your Intake of Proteins

Having achieved a low-carbohydrate intake and an increased fat intake, you now need to check your protein intake. Proteins are essential components of your body since they help in the growth and repair of body tissues. In the absence of proteins, your body muscles will be weak, and this may affect your health at large.

Engage in Physical Exercise

When your body has a low number of carbohydrates and eventually initiates Ketosis, you will find that you will have a sluggish feeling anytime you exercise. To prevent your body from becoming lazy during Ketosis, you should incorporate a daily workout routine as you start your keto diet.

You can likewise evaluate how you are feeling to identify whether your body is into Ketosis.

Some individuals might experience "keto influenza." That can last for merely a couple of days or as much as a couple of weeks. It generally consists of signs consisting of headache, nausea, tiredness, sleeping disorders, irregularity, and irritation. Ensuring you remain consuming and hydrated with lots of electrolytes can assist in treating these signs quicker.

Other typical symptoms and signs to keep an eye out for consist of:

- Increased thirst and more regular urination.
- Keto breathes or fruity-smelling breath.
- Dry mouth.
- A decline in cravings.
- Weight reduction.

- Preliminary weak point and tiredness (this must ultimately decrease)
- Insufficient sleep disturbances
- Increased energy, psychological clearness, and focus

Chapter 2: Keto Diet for Women Over 50

Metabolism

As women age, their metabolism naturally slows down by approximately 50 calories per day. This means that you need to consume fewer calories if you maintain the same level of activity.

During menopause, when estrogen levels decrease, fat storage is promoted around. While you may have struggled your entire life with weight gain in your hips and thighs, this new fat in your belly area is not only more difficult to lose but brings with it additional health risks to your heart and organs.

Why Keto

The premise of this guidebook is to provide women over 50 with a healthy alternative way of eating to remain healthy and increase their chances of longevity. It also assumes that you do not suffer from health issues that may prohibit you from eating certain foods and from exercising.

While the keto way of eating is beneficial for anyone at any age, for women of 50, it can have dramatic and even life-saving benefits.

- Abdominal fat. Yes, I said it! There is no denying that as we age, we all tend to get a little more around the middle. Otherwise known as visceral fat, it is not only difficult to lose but increases the risk of health problems.

Keto increases fat burning, specifically targeting abdominal fat.

- Insulin sensitivity. As you consume carbohydrates, they are naturally converted into glucose, which is then transported by insulin throughout the body. With age, the body's sensitivity to insulin decreases, increasing the risk of Type 2 diabetes.

Keto increases insulin sensitivity and thereby reduces the risk of developing diabetes.

- Reduced inflammation. Inflammation is part of the body's natural healing process. As women age, it can occur more frequently, causing pain and discomfort.

Keto, as a high-fat diet, can have a dramatic impact on reducing inflammation.

- Brain function. As the female body ages, reduced hormone levels can cause women to experience mood swings, memory loss, difficulty concentrating, and can even trigger depression and anxiety.

The keto diet provides the brain with an alternate source of fuel in ketones.

- Improved cardiovascular health. Increased levels of triglycerides and "bad" cholesterol puts women over 50 at a higher risk of heart disease.

Keto is a low-carbohydrate diet that reduces triglycerides and increases "good" cholesterol, thereby reducing the risk of heart disease.

- Decreased blood pressure. Although it is common for women to have lower blood pressure levels than men, it does tend to increase with age. High blood pressure brings additional risks of heart disease, stroke, and even kidney disease.

Keto is a low-carbohydrate diet, can help to reduce blood pressure.

- Muscle loss. As women age, they naturally tend to lose muscle mass, which further reduces metabolism. Muscle loss can also prevent a woman from being physically active.

Keto provides a higher amount of protein, which is critical for muscle mass and to prevent loss.

- Increased bone density. Women are prone to lose bone mass, which can lead to osteoporosis, the key factor in bone weakness and fracture.

Keto can help improve bone strength and density with its high levels of calcium-rich leafy greens.
Keto diet is not only beneficial to women for weight loss. However, it has so many added benefits that not implementing keto as a lifestyle may be detrimental to the health of a woman over 50!

It is important to note that you should consult with your physician before starting a new diet and exercise regimen. Nothing contained in this guidebook should be considered medical advice, nor is it a guarantee that you will reap the benefits as described.

By considering keto to be a lifestyle, not a diet, you will be well on your way to weight loss and living a healthier lifestyle.

How to Start after 50?

As you get older, it gets harder for you to make decisions. But if you want to gain more energy and stay fit in your 50s, you should try the Keto diet. Below, you'll find the complete guide for beginners. Here are some simple steps that'll help you start the low-carbohydrate diet successfully:

Reduce Your Carbohydrate Intake to 20-30 Grams per Day

This is the crucial rule of the Keto diet because only if the carbohydrate levels are very-very low, your body can produce ketones. However, this rule doesn't refer to fiber that can be highly effective in stimulating ketone levels.

Keep Moderate Protein Consumption

Here, 'moderate' means no less than 25 percent of calories. For example, if your weight is 70 kilos, you can eat about 100-130 g of protein per day. You should know that consuming too much protein can stop ketosis because the body can turn excess protein into glucose.

Consume Enough Fat

The essence of this diet is increasing fat intake. So, you add enough fat to your meals to feel full. Just try not to overeat and not to eat when you don't feel hungry.

Regulate Sleep Patterns

People over 50 should sleep 8-9 hours per night. Keep that in mind, as sleep deprivation may cause slower ketosis.

Stay Active

Inserting any kind of physical activity when sticking to the Keto diet may also speed up ketosis. This is not a requirement. However, visiting a sports gym can have a positive effect not only on physical but also mental health.

The Keto diet is quite easy to do. However, for most middle-aged people, it can be rather challenging to adapt to it at first. According to studies, it commonly takes about 3 weeks to make a new habit. That's why you should be patient if you want to reach your goal.

Chapter 3: Which Foods Should I Eat on a Keto Diet

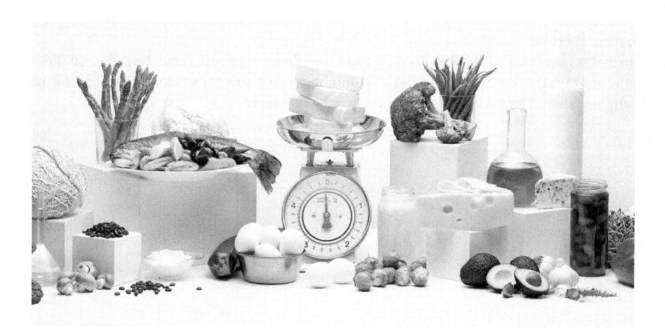

To help you, here is a list of items to get when grocery-shopping on the keto diet. Each product on the list is perfectly healthy and beneficial for a woman of 50 years who is on a keto diet.

Meat and Poultry

- Chicken
- Beef
- Pork
- Lamb
- Turkey
- Veal
- Bacon
- Organ meats

Seafood

When it comes to seafood, you also have an excellent list. You can buy and cook a lot of delicious dishes from:

- Lobster
- Shrimp
- Octopus
- Salmon
- Tuna
- Oysters
- Mussels
- Squid
- Scallops
- Crab

Vegetables

Only low-carbohydrates and non-starchy veggies can be eaten by the people who go on the Keto diet. This means that you can add the following vegetables:

- Avocados
- Tomatoes
- Cucumbers
- Zucchini
- Radishes
- Mushrooms
- Eggplant
- Celery
- Bell peppers
- Herbs
- Asparagus
- Kohlrabi
- Mustard
- Spinach
- Lettuce
- Kale
- Brussel sprouts

Dairy Products

You should be careful with dairy. Not all dairy food can be useful for you if you want to stick to the Keto diet. Here are the products you can buy and cook:

- Eggs
- Butter and ghee
- Heavy cream and whipping cream
- Sour cream
- Unflavored Greek yogurt
- Cottage cheese
- Hard, semi-hard, soft, and cream cheeses

Berries

Unfortunately, most fruits have high levels of carbohydrates and can't be included on the Keto diet. However, you can consume:

- Blackberries
- Raspberries
- Strawberries
- Blueberries

Nuts and Seeds

A lot of experts recommend paying attention to nuts and seeds that are high-fat and low-carbohydrates. You can add such nuts and seeds to your dishes as:

- Almond Pecans
- Walnuts
- Hazelnuts
- Brazil nuts
- Pumpkin seeds
- Sesame seeds
- Chia seeds
- Flaxseed

Coconut and Olive Oils

To cook tasty fatty dishes, you need oil. Coconut and olive oils have unique properties that make them suitable for a Keto diet. These oils are rich in fat and boost ketone production. Moreover, they can be used for salad dressing and adding to cooked dishes.

Low-Carbohydrate Drinks

- Unsweetened coffee
- Tea
- Dark chocolate
- Cocoa

Chapter 4: What to Avoid in The Keto Diet

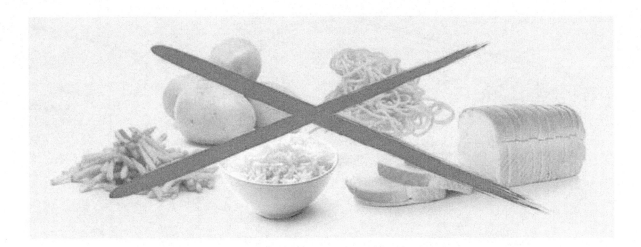

Because the diet is ketogenic, that means you should avoid carbohydrate-rich foods. Some of the food you avoid is even healthy, but it just contains too many carbohydrates. Here is a list of typical food you should limit or avoid altogether.

- Grains (like oatmeal, pasta, bulgur, corn, wheat, buckwheat, rice, etc.)
- Low-fat dairy (fat-free yogurt, skim milk, skim Mozzarella, etc.)
- Most fruits (melon, watermelon, apples, peaches, bananas, grapes, oranges, plums, grapefruits, mangos, cherries, pineapples, pears, etc.)
- Starchy veggies (potatoes, beets, turnips, parsnips, etc.)
- Grain foods (pasta, popcorn, muesli, cereal, bagels, bread, etc.)
- Some oils (soyabean oil, grapeseed oil, sunflower oil, peanut oil, canola oil)
- Typical snack foods (crackers, potato chips, etc.)
- Trans fat (margarine)
- Sweets (candies, buns, pastries, cakes, chocolate, puddings, cookies)
- Sweeteners and added sugars (corn syrup, cane sugar, honey, agave nectar, etc.)
- Sweetened drinks (sweetened coffee and tea, juice, soda, smoothies)
- Alcohol (sweet wines, cider, beer, etc.)

Chapter 5: Breakfast

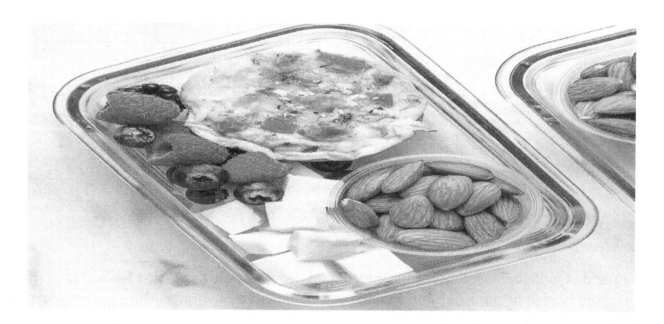

Cheesy Breakfast Muffins

Preparation Time: 15 minutes
Cooking Time: 12 minutes
Servings: 2
Ingredients:

- 2 tbsp. melted butter
- 3/4 tbsp. baking powder
- 1 cup almond flour
- 1 large egg, lightly beaten
-
- 2 oz. cream cheese mixed with 2 tbsp. heavy whipping cream
- A handful of shredded Mexican blend cheese

Directions:

1. Preheat the oven to 400°F. Grease 2 muffin tin cups with melted butter and set aside.
2. Combine the baking powder and almond flour in a bowl. Stir well and set aside.
3. Stir together four tbsp. melted butter, eggs, shredded cheese, and cream cheese in a separate bowl.
4. The egg and the dry mixture must be combined using a hand mixer to beat until it is creamy and well blended.
5. The mixture must be scooped into the greased muffin cups evenly.

Nutrition:

- Net Carbohydrates: 2 g
- Protein: 9.5 g
- Fat: 15.6g
- Calories: 214

Bagels with Cheese

Preparation Time: 10 minutes
Cooking Time: 15 minutes
Servings: 2
Ingredients:

- 2.5 cups mozzarella cheese
- 1 tsp. baking powder
- 3 oz. cream cheese
- 1.5 cups almond flour
- 2 eggs

Directions:

1. Shred the mozzarella and combine with the flour, baking powder, and cream cheese. Microwave for one minute. Mix.
2. Cool and put the eggs. Break into six parts and shape into round bagels.
3. Bake for 12 to 15 minutes. Serve.

Nutrition:

- Net Carbohydrates: 8 g
- Protein: 19 g
- Fat: 31 g
- Calories: 374

Bacon & Avocado Omelet

Preparation Time: 5 minutes
Cooking Time: 5 minutes
Servings: 2
Ingredients:

- 2 slice crispy bacon
- 2 large organic eggs
- 5 cup freshly grated parmesan cheese
- 2 tbsp ghee or coconut oil or butter
- half of 1 small avocado

Directions:

1. Prepare the bacon to your liking and set aside. Combine the eggs, parmesan cheese, and your choice of finely chopped herbs. Warm a skillet and add the butter/ghee to melt using the medium-high heat setting. When the pan is hot, whisk and add the eggs.
2. Prepare the omelet, working it towards the middle of the pan for about 30 seconds. When firm, flip, and cook it for another 30 seconds. Arrange the omelet on a plate and garnish it with the crunched bacon bits. Serve with sliced avocado.

Nutrition:

- Net Carbohydrates: 3.3 g
- Protein: 30 g
- Fat: 63 g
- Calories: 71

Keto Fruit Cereal

Preparation Time: 20 minutes
Cooking Time: 5 minutes
Servings: 2
Ingredients:

- 1 cup of coconut flakes
- ½ cup of sliced strawberries
- ¼ cup of sliced raspberries

Directions:

1. Preheat oven to 300 degrees F.
2. Prepare a baking tray with parchment paper
3. Slice the berries into small bits.
4. Spread the coconut flakes on the tray, bake for 5 minutes until brown from the edges.
5. Take out the baked coconut cereals, let them cool.
6. Then, add in sliced raspberries and strawberries.
7. Enjoy with almond milk.

Nutrition:

- Net Carbohydrates: 4g
- Protein: 19g
- Fat: 44g
- Calories: 201

Brunch BLT Wrap

Preparation Time: 5 minutes
Cooking Time: 15 minutes
Servings: 2
Ingredients:

- 2 bacon slices
- 2 Romaine lettuce leaves
- 0.25 cup tomatoes
- 1tbsp. Mayo
- Pepper

Directions:

1. Cook the bacon until crispy in a skillet. Spread mayonnaise on one side of the lettuce.
2. Add the bacon and tomato. Roll it up and serve.

Nutrition:

- Net Carbohydrates: 2 g
- Protein: 8 g
- Fat: 24 g
- Calories: 256

Cheesy Bacon & Egg Cups

Preparation Time: 10 minutes
Cooking Time: 20 minutes
Servings: 2
Ingredients:

- 2 slice bacon
- 2 large eggs
- 0.25 cup cheese
- 1 spinach
- pepper

Directions:

1. Set the oven setting to 400º Fahrenheit. Cook the bacon in medium-heat. Grease muffin tins. Put the slice of bacon. Mix the eggs and combine with the spinach. Add the batter to tins and sprinkle with cheese. Put salt and pepper. Bake for 15 minutes. Serve.

Nutrition:

- Net Carbohydrates: 1 g
- Protein: 8 g
- Fat: 7 g
- Calories: 101

Coconut Keto Porridge

Preparation Time: 15 minutes
Cooking Time: 10 minutes
Servings: 2
Ingredients:

- 4 tbsp. coconut cream
- 1 pinch ground psyllium husk powder
- 1 tbsp. coconut flour
- 1 flaxseed egg
- 1oz. coconut butter

Directions:

1. Toss all of the mixtures in a small pan, cook on low heat. Serve.

Nutrition:

- Net Carbohydrates: 5.4 g
- Protein: 10.1 g
- Fat: 22.8 g
- Calories: 401

Mexican Scrambled Eggs

Preparation Time: 5 minutes
Cooking Time: 5 minutes
Servings: 2
Ingredients:

- 1/2 tsp salt
- 3 eggs
- 1/2 scallion, chopped
- 1/2 medium tomato, chopped
- 1 pickled jalapeño, chopped
- 1 ½ oz. shredded cheddar cheese
- 1 tbsp butter
- 1/2 tsp salt
- ½ tsp ground black pepper

Directions:

1. Place a large skillet pan over medium-high heat, add butter and when it melts, add scallion, tomato, and jalapeno and cook for 3 minutes or until beginning to soften.
2. Meanwhile, crack eggs in a bowl and whisk until beaten.
3. Pour the egg mixture into the pan, scramble eggs for 2 minutes, then sprinkle cheese on top and season with salt and black pepper.
4. Serve straight away.

Nutrition:

- Net Carbohydrates: 2g
- Protein: 14g
- Fat: 12g
- Calories: 229

Coconut Porridge

Preparation Time: 5 minutes
Cooking Time: 10 minutes
Servings: 2
Ingredients

- 2 eggs, beaten
- 2 tbsp coconut flour
- 1/8 tsp. salt
- 1/8 tsp. psyllium husk powder grounded
- 2 oz. butter
- 8 tbsp coconut cream

Directions:

1. Crack eggs in a bowl, add flour, salt, and Psyllium husk, and whisk until combined.
2. Place a saucepan over low heat, add butter and when it melts, whisk in coconut cream.
3. Then slowly whisk in egg mixture until a smooth and creamy mixture comes together.
4. Divide porridge evenly between two bowls and serve with berries.

Nutrition:

- Net Carbohydrates: 4g
- Protein: 9g
- Fat: 49g
- Calories: 486

Cauliflower Hash Browns

Preparation Time: 10 minutes
Cooking Time: 30 minutes
Servings: 2
Ingredients:

- ½ lb. cauliflower, grated
- 2 eggs
- ¼ white onion, grated
- ½ tsp salt
- ¼ tsp ground black pepper
- 2 oz. butter, for frying

Directions:

1. Place grated cauliflower in a bowl, add remaining ingredients and stir until mixed, let the mixture rest for 10 minutes.
2. Then place a skillet pan over medium heat, add butter and when it melts, lower the heat and place scoops of the cauliflower mixture.
3. Flatten each mixture into 3 to 4-inch patties and fry for 4 to 5 minutes per side or until nicely golden brown and cooked.
4. Serve straight away.

Nutrition:

- Net Carbohydrates: 5g
- Protein: 7g
- Fat: 26g
- Calories: 282

Cream Cheese Eggs

Preparation Time: 5 minutes
Cooking Time: 5 minutes
Servings: 2
Ingredients:

- 1 tbsp. Butter
- 2 Eggs
- 2 tbsp. Soft cream cheese with chives

Directions:

1. Warm-up a skillet and melt the butter. Whisk the eggs with the cream cheese.
2. Cook until done. Serve.

Nutrition:

- Net Carbohydrates: 3 g
- Protein: 15 g
- Fat: 31 g
- Calories: 341

Creamy Basil Baked Sausage

Preparation Time: 5 minutes
Cooking Time: 5 minutes
Servings: 2
Ingredients:

- 3 lb. Italian sausage
- 8 oz. Cream cheese
- 0.25 cup Heavy cream
- 0.25 cup Basil pesto
- 8 oz. Mozzarella

Directions:

1. Set the oven at 400° Fahrenheit.
2. Put the sausage to the dish and bake for 30 minutes. Combine the heavy cream, pesto, and cream cheese. Pour the sauce over the casserole and top it off with the cheese.
3. Bake for 10 minutes. Serve.

Nutrition:

- Net Carbohydrates: 4 g
- Protein: 23 g
- Fat: 23 g
- Calories: 316

Ricotta Pancakes

Preparation Time: 10 minutes
Cooking Time: 20 minutes
Servings: 2
Ingredients

- 2 organic eggs
- ½ cup ricotta cheese
- ¼ cup unsweetened vanilla whey protein powder
- ½ tsp. organic baking powder
- Pinch of salt
- ½ tsp. liquid stevia
- 2 tbsp. unsalted butter

Directions

1. In a blender, add all the ingredients and pulse until well combined.
2. In a wok, melt butter over medium heat.
3. Add the desired amount of the mixture and spread it evenly.
4. Cook for about 2–3 minutes or until the bottom becomes golden brown.
5. Flip and cook for about 1–2 minutes or until golden brown.
6. Repeat with the remaining mixture.
7. Serve warm.

Nutrition:

- Net Carbohydrates: 2.7 g
- Fat: 23 g
- Protein: 14.6 g
- Calories: 184

Yogurt Waffles

Preparation Time: 15 minutes
Cooking Time: 25 minutes
Servings: 2
Ingredients:

- ½ cup golden flax seeds meal
- ½ cup plus 3 tbsp. almond flour
- 1-1½ tbsp. granulated erythritol
- 1 tbsp. unsweetened vanilla whey protein powder
- ½ tsp. organic powder
- ¼ tsp. xanthan gum
- Salt, as required
- 1 large organic egg, white and yolk separated
- 1 organic whole egg
- 2 tbsp. unsweetened almond milk
- 1½ tbsp. unsalted butter
- 3 oz. plain Greek yogurt
- ¼ tsp. baking soda

Directions:

1. Preheat the waffle iron and then grease it.
2. In a large bowl, add the flour, erythritol, protein powder, baking soda, baking powder, xanthan gum, and salt, and mix until well combined.
3. In a second small bowl, add the egg white and beat until stiff peaks form.
4. In a third bowl, add 2 egg yolks, whole egg, almond milk, butter, and yogurt, and beat until well combined.
5. Place egg mixture into the bowl of the flour mixture and mix until well combined.
6. Gently fold in the beaten egg whites.
7. Place ¼ cup of the mixture into preheated waffle iron and cook for about 4–5 minutes or until golden brown.
8. Repeat with the remaining mixture.
9. Serve warm.

Nutrition:

- Net Carbohydrates: 3.2 g
- Fat: 15 g
- Protein: 8.4 g
- Calories: 250

Baked Eggs in the Avocado

Preparation Time: 10 minutes
Cooking Time: 20 minutes
Servings: 2
Ingredients:

- ½ Avocado
- 1 Egg
- 1tbsp.Olive oil
- 0.5cup Shredded cheddar cheese

Directions:

1. Heat the oven to reach 425° Fahrenheit.
2. Remove the avocado flesh. Drizzle with oil and put the eggs.
3. Sprinkle with cheese and bake for 15 to 16 minutes. Serve.

Nutrition:

- Net Carbohydrates: 3 g
- Protein: 21 g
- Fat: 52 g
- Calories: 452

French Toast

Preparation Time: 25 minutes
Cooking Time: 10 minutes
Servings: 2
Ingredients
For Mug bread

- 2 tbsp Almond flour
- 2 tbsp Coconut flour
- 1½ tsp Baking powder
- 1/16 tsp Salt
- 1 tsp Butter
- 2 Eggs
- 1 tbsp Heavy whipping cream

For Batter

- 2 Eggs
- 1/16 tsp Salt
- tsp Ground cinnamon
- 2 tbsp Heavy whipping cream
- 2 tbsp Butter

Directions:

1. Take a heatproof mug, grease it with butter, then add all flours, baking powder, and salt and stir until mixed.
2. Crack eggs in it, then add cream and whisk until smooth batter comes together.
3. Place the mug into the microwave and cook for 2 minutes at high heat setting or until bread is cooked through, check bread by inserting a toothpick into the center, and it should come out clean.
4. When done, remove the mug from the oven and let cool for 15 minutes.
5. Then take out the bread and slice it in half.

6. Prepare batter and for this, crack eggs in a bowl, add salt, cinnamon, and cream and whisk until smooth.
7. Pour this mixture over the bread slices and let soak completely, turning slices a few times.
8. Then place a skillet pan over medium heat, add butter and when it melts, add bread slices and cook for 3 to 4 minutes per side or until nicely golden brown and crispy.
9. Serve straight away with berries.

Nutrition:

- Net Carbohydrates: 4g
- Protein: 15g
- Fat: 37g
- Calories: 416

Chapter 6: Soups and First Courses

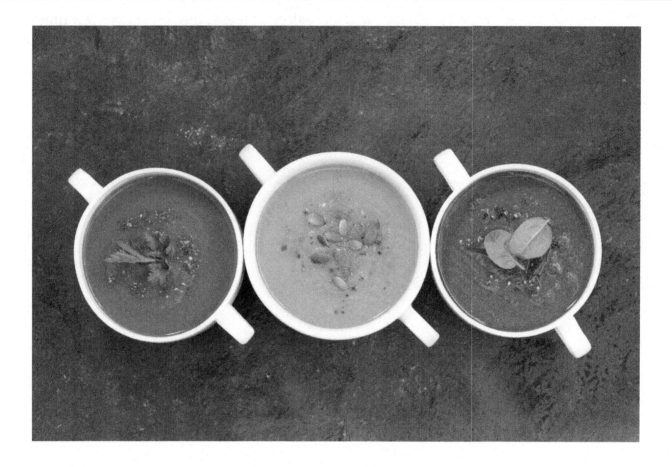

Spiced Jalapeno Bites with Tomato

Preparation Time: 10 minutes
Cooking Time: 0 minutes
Servings: 2
Ingredients:

- 1 cup turkey ham, chopped
- 1/4 jalapeño pepper, minced
- 1/4 cup mayonnaise
- 1/3 tbsp. Dijon mustard
- chopped
- 4 tomatoes, sliced
- Salt and black pepper to taste
- 1 tbsp. parsley,

Directions:

1. In a bowl, mix the turkey ham, jalapeño pepper, mayo, mustard, salt, and pepper.
2. Spread out the tomato slices on four serving plates, then top each plate with a spoonful of turkey ham mixture.
3. Serve garnished with chopped parsley.

Nutrition:

- Net Carbohydrates: 4.1 g
- Protein:18.9 g
- Fat: 14.1g
- Calories: 250

Coconut Crab Cakes

Preparation Time: 20 minutes
Cooking Time: 25 minutes
Servings: 2
Ingredients:

- 1 tbsp. of minced garlic
- 2 pasteurized eggs
- 2 tsp. of coconut oil
- 3/4 cup of coconut flakes
- 3/4 cup chopped of spinach
- 1/4-lb. crabmeat
- 1/4 cup of chopped leek
- 1/2 cup extra virgin olive oil
- 1/2 tsp. of pepper
- 1/4 onion diced
- Salt

Directions:

1. Pour the crabmeat into a bowl, then add in the coconut flakes and mix well.
2. Whisk eggs in a bowl, then mix in leek and spinach.
3. Season the egg mixture with pepper, two pinches of salt, and garlic.
4. Then, pour the eggs into the crab and stir well.
5. Preheat a pan, heat extra virgin olive, and fry the crab evenly from each side until golden brown. Remove from pan and serve hot.

Nutrition:

- Net Carbohydrates: 4.1 g
- Protein: 8.9g
- Fat: 9.5g
- Calories: 254

Tuna Cakes

Preparation Time: 15 minutes
Cooking Time: 10 minutes
Servings: 2
Ingredients:

- 1 (15-oz.) can water-packed tuna, drained
- 1/2 celery stalk, chopped
- 2 tbsp. fresh parsley, chopped
- 1 tsp. fresh dill, chopped
- 2 tbsp. walnuts, chopped
- 2 tbsp. mayonnaise
- 1 organic egg, beaten
- 1 tbsp. butter
- 3 cups lettuce

Directions:

1. For burgers: Add all ingredients (except the butter and lettuce) to a bowl and mix until well combined.
2. Make two equal-sized patties from the mixture.
3. Melt some butter and cook the patties for about 2–3 minutes.
4. Carefully flip the side and cook for about 2–3 minutes.
5. Divide the lettuce onto serving plates.
6. Top each plate with one burger and serve.

Nutrition:

- Net Carbohydrates: 3.8 g
- Protein: 11.5g
- Fat: 12.5g
- Calories: 267

Creamed Spinach

Preparation Time: 10 minutes
Cooking Time: 15 minutes
Servings: 2
Ingredients:

- 2 tbsp. unsalted butter
- 1 small yellow onion, chopped
- 1 cup cream cheese, softened
- 2 (10-oz.) packages frozen spinach, thawed and squeezed dry
- 2–3 tbsp. water
- Salt and ground black pepper, as required
- 1 tsp. fresh lemon juice

Directions:

1. Melt some butter and sauté the onion for about 6–8 minutes.
2. Add the cream cheese and cook for about 2 minutes or until melted completely.
3. Stir in the water and spinach and cook for about 4–5 minutes.
4. Stir in the salt, black pepper, and lemon juice, and remove from heat.
5. Serve immediately.

Nutrition:

- Net Carbohydrates: 2.1 g
- Protein: 4.2g
- Fat: 9.5g
- Calories: 214

Tempura Zucchini with Cream Cheese Dip

Preparation Time: 15 minutes
Cooking Time: 15 minutes
Servings: 2
Ingredients:
Tempura zucchinis:

- 1 1/2 cups (200 g) almond flour
- 2 tbsp. heavy cream
- 1 tsp. salt
- 2 tbsp. olive oil + extra for frying
- 1 1/4 cups (300 ml) water
- 1/2 tbsp. sugar-free maple syrup
- 2 large zucchinis, cut into 1-inch thick strips

Cream cheese dip:

- 8 oz cream cheese, room temperature
- 1/2 cup (113 g) sour cream
- 1 tsp. taco seasoning
- 1 scallion, chopped
- 1 green chili, deseeded and minced

Directions:
Tempura zucchinis:

1. In a bowl, mix the almond flour, heavy cream, salt, peanut oil, water, and maple syrup.
2. Dredge the zucchini strips in the mixture until well-coated.

3. Heat about four tbsp. of olive oil in a non-stick skillet.
4. Working in batches, use tongs to remove the zucchinis (draining extra liquid) into the oil.
5. Fry per side for 1 to 2 minutes and remove the zucchinis onto a paper towel-lined plate to drain grease.
6. Enjoy the zucchinis.

Cream cheese dip:

1. In a bowl or container, the cream cheese, taco seasoning, sour cream, scallion, and green chili must be mixed,
2. Serve the tempura zucchinis with the cream cheese dip.

Nutrition:

- Net Carbohydrates: 4.1 g
- Protein: 5.1g
- Fat: 8.4g
- Calories: 316

Quinoa Salad with Fresh Mint and Parsley

Preparation Time: 10 minutes
Cooking Time: 15 minutes
Servings: 2
Ingredients:

- 2 cups of quinoa
- 1/2 cup of almond nut
- 3 tbsp. of fresh parsley (chopped)
- 1/2 cup of chopped green onions
- 3 tbsp. of chopped fresh mint
- 3 tbsp. of olive oil
- 2 tbsp. of lemon juice
- 1 tsp. of garlic salt
- 1/2 tsp. of salt and pepper

Directions:

1. Place a saucepan on high heat.
2. Add the quinoa and water and just let it boil for around 15 minutes, then reduce the heat and drain.
3. Pour the drained quinoa into a large bowl, add the parsley, almond nuts, and mint.
4. In a bowl or container, add the olive oil, garlic salt, and lemon juice together.
5. Whisk the mixture well until it's well combined and pour over the quinoa.
6. Combine the mixture well until everything is well dispersed.
7. Add the salt and black pepper to taste.
8. Place the quinoa mixture bowl in the refrigerator.

Nutrition:

- Net Carbohydrates: 2.1 g
- Protein: 9.3g
- Fat: 8.4g
- Calories: 241

Coconut Soup

Preparation Time: 15 minutes
Cooking Time: 35 minutes
Servings: 2
Ingredients:

- 1½ cups of coconut milk
- 4 cups chicken stock
- 1 tsp fried lemongrass
- 3 lime leaves
- 4 Thai chilies, dried and chopped
- 1-inch fresh ginger, peeled and grated
- 1 cup fresh cilantro, chopped
- Salt and ground black pepper to taste
- 1 tbsp fish sauce
- 1 tbsp coconut oil
- 2 tbsp mushrooms, chopped
- 4 oz shrimp, peeled and deveined
- 2 tbsp onion, chopped
- 1 tbsp fresh cilantro, chopped
- Juice from 1 lime

Directions:

1. In a medium pot, combine coconut milk, chicken stock, lemongrass, and lime leaves.
2. Preheat the pot on medium heat.
3. Add Thai chilies, ginger, cilantro, salt, and pepper, stir and bring to simmer—Cook for 20 minutes.
4. Strain the soup and return liquid to the pot.
5. Heat the soup over medium heat.
6. Add fish sauce, coconut oil, mushrooms, shrimp, and onion. Stir well—Cook for 10 minutes.
7. Add cilantro and lime juice, stir. Set aside for 10 minutes.
8. Serve.

Nutrition:

- Net Carbohydrates: 7.9g
- Protein: 11.8g
- Fat: 33.8g
- Calories: 448

Broccoli Soup

Preparation Time: 12 minutes
Cooking Time: 35 minutes
Servings: 2
Ingredients:

- 2 cloves garlic
- 1 medium white onion
- 1 tbsp butter
- 2 cups of water
- 2 cups vegetable stock
- 1 cup heavy cream
- Salt and ground black pepper to taste
- ½ tsp paprika
- 1½ cups broccoli, divided into florets
- 1 cup cheddar cheese

Directions:

1. Peel and mince garlic. Peel and chop the onion.
2. Preheat the pot on medium heat, add butter and melt it.
3. Add garlic and onion and sauté for 5 minutes, stirring occasionally.
4. Pour in water, vegetable stock, heavy cream, and add pepper, salt, and paprika.
5. Stir and bring to a boil.
6. Add broccoli and simmer for 25 minutes.
7. After that, transfer the soup mixture to a food processor and blend well.
8. Grate cheddar cheese and add to a food processor, blend again.
9. Serve soup hot.

Nutrition:

- Net Carbohydrates: 6.8g
- Protein: 10.9g
- Fat: 33.8g
- Calories: 348

Simple Tomato Soup

Preparation Time: 15 minutes
Cooking Time: 10 minutes
Servings: 2
Ingredients:

- 4 cups canned tomato soup
- 2 tbsp apple cider vinegar
- 1 tsp dried oregano
- 4 tbsp butter
- 2 tsp turmeric
- 2 oz red hot sauce
- Salt and ground black pepper to taste
- 4 tbsp olive oil
- 8 bacon strips, cooked and crumbled
- 4 oz fresh basil leaves, chopped
- 4 oz green onions, chopped

Directions:

1. Pour tomato soup into the pot and preheat on medium heat. Bring to a boil.
2. Add vinegar, oregano, butter, turmeric, hot sauce, salt, black pepper, and olive oil. Stir well.
3. Simmer the soup for 5 minutes.
4. Serve soup topped with crumbled bacon, green onion, and basil.

Nutrition:

- Net Carbohydrates: 9g
- Protein: 11.7g
- Fat: 33.8
- Calories: 397

Green Soup

Preparation Time: 12 minutes
Cooking Time: 15 minutes
Servings: 2
Ingredients:

- 2 cloves garlic
- 1 white onion
- 1 cauliflower head
- 2 oz butter
- 1 bay leaf, crushed
- 1 cup spinach leaves
- ½ cup watercress
- 4 cups vegetable stock
- Salt and ground black pepper to taste
- 1 cup of coconut milk
- ½ cup parsley for serving

Directions:

1. Peel and mince garlic. Peel and dice onion.
2. Divide cauliflower into florets.
3. Preheat the pot on medium-high heat, add butter and melt it.
4. Add onion and garlic, stir, and sauté for 4 minutes.
5. Add cauliflower and bay leaf, stir and cook for 5 minutes.
6. Add spinach and watercress, stir and cook for another 3 minutes.
7. Pour in vegetable stock—season with salt and black pepper. Stir and bring to a boil.
8. Pour in coconut milk and stir well. Take off heat.
9. Use an immersion blender to blend well.
10. Top with parsley and serve hot.

Nutrition:

- Net Carbohydrates: 4.89g
- Protein: 6.97g
- Fat: 35.1
- Calories: 227

Sausage and Peppers Soup

Preparation Time: 15 minutes
Cooking Time: 1 hour 15 minutes
Servings: 2
Ingredients:

- 1 tbsp avocado oil
- 2 lbs. pork sausage meat
- Salt and ground black pepper to taste
- 1 green bell pepper, seeded and chopped
- 5 oz canned jalapeños, chopped
- 5 oz canned tomatoes, chopped
- 1¼ cup spinach
- 4 cups beef stock
- 1 tsp Italian seasoning
- 1 tbsp cumin
- 1 tsp onion powder
- 1 tsp garlic powder
- 1 tbsp chili powder

Directions:

1. Preheat pot with avocado oil on medium heat.
2. Put sausage meat in pot and brown for 3 minutes on all sides.
3. Add salt, black pepper, and green bell pepper and continue to cook for 3 minutes.
4. Add jalapeños and tomatoes, stir well, and cook for 2 minutes more.
5. Toss spinach and stir again, close the lid and cook for 7 minutes.
6. Pour in beef stock, Italian seasoning, cumin, onion powder, chili powder, garlic powder, salt, and black pepper, stir well. Close lid again. Cook for 30 minutes.
7. When time is up, uncover the pot and simmer for 15 minutes more.
8. Serve hot.

Nutrition:

- Net Carbohydrates: 3.99g
- Protein: 25.8g
- Fat: 44.5g
- Calories: 531

Avocado Soup

Preparation Time: 12 minutes
Cooking Time: 15 minutes
Servings: 2
Ingredients:

- 2 tbsp butter
- 2 scallions, chopped
- 3 cups chicken stock
- 2 avocados, pitted, peeled, and chopped
- Salt and ground black pepper to taste
- ⅔ cup heavy cream

Directions:

1. Preheat the pot on medium heat, add butter and melt it.
2. Toss scallions, stir, and sauté for 2 minutes.
3. Pour in 2 ½ cups stock and bring to simmer—Cook for 3 minutes.
4. Meanwhile, peel and chop avocados.
5. Place avocado, ½ cup of stock, cream, salt, and pepper in a blender and blend well.
6. Add avocado mixture to the pot and mix well—Cook for 2 minutes.
7. Sprinkle with more salt and pepper, stir.
8. Serve hot.

Nutrition:

- Net Carbohydrates: 5.9g
- Protein: 5.8g
- Fat: 22.9g
- Calories: 329

Avocado and Bacon Soup

Preparation Time: 15 minutes
Cooking Time: 15 minutes
Servings: 2
Ingredients:

- 1-quart chicken stock
- 2 avocados, pitted
- ⅓ cup fresh cilantro, chopped
- 1 tsp garlic powder
- Salt and ground black pepper to taste
- Juice of ½ lime
- ½ lb. bacon, cooked and chopped

Directions:

1. Pour chicken stock in a pot and bring to a boil over medium-high heat.
2. Meanwhile, peeled and chopped avocados.
3. Place avocados, cilantro, garlic powder, salt, black pepper, and lime juice in the blender or food processor and blend well.
4. Add the avocado mixture in boiling stock and stir well.
5. Add bacon and season with salt and pepper to taste.
6. Stir and simmer for 3-4 minutes on medium heat.
7. Serve hot.

Nutrition:

- Net Carbohydrates: 5.98g
- Protein: 16.8g
- Fat: 22.8g
- Calories: 298

Roasted Bell Peppers Soup

Preparation Time: 15 minutes
Cooking Time: 20 minutes
Servings: 2
Ingredients:

- 1 medium white onion
- 2 cloves garlic
- 2 celery stalks
- 12 oz roasted bell peppers, seeded
- 2 tbsp olive oil
- Salt and ground black pepper to taste
- 1-quart chicken stock
- 2/3 cup water
- 1/4 cup Parmesan cheese, grated
- 2/3 cup heavy cream

Directions:

1. Peel and chop onion and garlic. Chop celery and bell pepper.
2. Preheat pot with oil on medium heat.
3. Put garlic, onion, celery, salt, and pepper in the pot, stir and sauté for 8 minutes.
4. Pour in chicken stock and water. Add bell peppers and stir.
5. Bring to a boil, close the lid, and simmer for 5 minutes. Reduce heat if needed.

6. When time is up, blend soup using an immersion blender.
7. Add cream and season with salt and pepper to taste. Take off heat.
8. Serve hot with grated cheese.

Nutrition:
- Net Carbohydrates: 3.9g
- Protein: 5.9g
- Fat: 12.9g
- Calories: 180

Healthy Celery Soup

Preparation Time: 10 minutes
Cooking Time: 20 minutes
Servings: 2
Ingredients:
- 3 cups celery, chopped
- 1 cup vegetable broth
- 5 oz cream cheese
- 1 1/2 tbsp. fresh basil, chopped
- 1/4 cup onion, chopped
- 1 tbsp. garlic, chopped
- 1 tbsp. olive oil
- 1/4 tsp. pepper
- 1/2 tsp. salt

Directions:
1. Heat some oil.
2. Add celery, onion, and garlic to the saucepan and sauté for 4-5 minutes or until softened.
3. Add broth and bring to a boil. Turn heat to low and simmer.
4. Add basil and cream cheese and stir until cheese is melted.
5. Season soup with pepper and salt.
6. Puree the soup until smooth.
7. Serve and enjoy.

Nutrition:
- Net Carbohydrates: 3.9 g
- Protein: 5.1g
- Fat: 5.4g
- Calories: 201

Creamy Asparagus Soup

Preparation Time: 10 minutes
Cooking Time: 15 minutes
Servings: 2
Ingredients:

- 2 lbs. asparagus, cut the ends, and chop into 1/2-inch pieces
- 2 tbsp. olive oil
- 3 garlic cloves, minced
- 2 oz parmesan cheese, grated
- 1/2 cup heavy cream
- 1/4 cup onion, chopped
- 4 cups vegetable stock
- Pepper
- Salt

Directions:

1. Heat olive oil in a large pot over medium heat.
2. Add onion to the pot and sauté until onion is softened.
3. Add asparagus and sauté for 2-3 minutes.
4. Add garlic and sauté for a minute. Season with pepper and salt.
5. Add stock and bring to a boil. Turn heat to low and simmer until asparagus is tender.
6. Remove pot from heat and puree the soup using an immersion blender until creamy.
7. Return pot on heat. Add cream and stir well and cook over medium heat until just soup is hot. Do not boil the soup.
8. Remove from heat. Add cheese and stir well.
9. Serve and enjoy.

Nutrition:

- Net Carbohydrates: 3.1 g
- Protein: 5.3g
- Fat: 8.4g
- Calories: 202

Chapter 7: Fish and Seafood

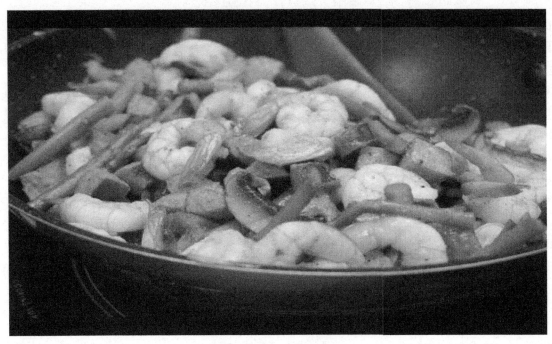

Shrimp Curry

Preparation Time: 15 minutes
Cooking Time: 20 minutes
Servings: 2
Ingredients:

- 2 tbsp. coconut oil
- 1/2 of yellow onion, minced
- 2 garlic cloves, minced
- 1 tsp. ground turmeric
- 1 tsp. ground cumin
- 1 tsp. paprika
- 1 (14-oz.) can unsweetened coconut milk
- 1 large tomato, chopped finely
- Salt, as required
- 1-lb. shrimp, peeled and deveined
- 2 tbsp. fresh cilantro, chopped

Directions:

1. The coconut oil must be melted in a wok medium heat and sauté the onion for about 5 minutes.
2. Add the garlic and spices, and sauté for about 1 minute.
3. Add the coconut milk, tomato, and salt, and bring to a gentle boil.
4. Let the curry simmer for about 10 minutes, stirring occasionally.
5. Stir in the shrimp and cilantro and simmer for about 4–5 minutes.

Nutrition:

- Net Carbohydrates: 4.1 g
- Protein: 14.1g
- Fat: 12.5g
- Calories: 354

Israeli Salmon Salad

Preparation Time: 10 minutes
Cooking Time: 0 minutes
Servings: 2
Ingredients:

- 1 cup flaked smoked salmon
- 1 tomato, chopped
- 1/2 small red onion, chopped
- 1 cucumber, chopped
- 6 tbsp. pitted green olives
- 1 avocado, chopped
- 2 tbsp. avocado oil
- 2 tbsp. almond oil
- 1 tbsp. plain vinegar
- Salt and black pepper to taste
- 1 cup crumbled feta cheese
- 1 cup grated cheddar cheese

Directions:

1. In a salad bowl, add the salmon, tomatoes, red onion, cucumber, green olives, and avocado. Mix well.
2. In a bowl, whisk the avocado oil, vinegar, salt, and black pepper.
3. Drizzle the dressing over the salad and toss well.
4. Sprinkle some feta cheese and serve the salad immediately.

Nutrition:

- Net Carbohydrates: 3.8 g
- Protein: 15.4g
- Fat: 11.4g
- Calories: 415

Parmesan-Garlic Salmon with Asparagus

Preparation Time: 10 minutes
Cooking Time: 15 minutes
Servings: 2
Ingredients:

- 2 (6-oz) salmon fillets, skin on
- Pink Himalayan salt
- Freshly ground black pepper
- 1 lb. fresh asparagus ends snapped off
- 3 tbsp. butter
- 2 garlic cloves, minced
- 1/4 cup grated Parmesan cheese

Directions:

1. Oven: 400°F.
2. Pat the salmon dry and season both sides with pink Himalayan salt and pepper.
3. Put the salmon and arrange the asparagus around the salmon.
4. Melt the butter. Add the minced garlic and stir until the garlic just begins to brown about 3 minutes.
5. Drizzle the garlic-butter sauce over the salmon and asparagus, and top both with the Parmesan cheese.
6. Bake until the salmon is cooked, and the asparagus is crisp-tender, about 12 minutes. You can switch the oven to broil at the end of cooking time to char the asparagus.
7. Serve hot.

Nutrition:

- Net Carbohydrates: 3.1 g
- Protein: 19.9g
- Fat: 14.1g
- Calories: 476

Spicy Shrimp Skewers

Preparation Time: 5 minutes
Cooking Time: 3-9 minutes
Servings: 2
Ingredients:

- 2 tbsp. Paprika
- 1/2 tbsp. Onion powder
- 1/2 tbsp. dried thyme, crushed
- 1-lb. shrimp, peeled and deveined
- 2 tbsp. Olive oil
- 1/2 tbsp. Red chili powder
- 1/2 tbsp. Garlic powder
- 1/2 tbsp. dried oregano, crushed
- 2 zucchinis, cut into 1/2-inch cubes

Directions:

1. Preheat the grill to medium-high heat.
2. In a bowl, mix spices and dried herbs.
3. In a large bowl, add shrimp, zucchini, oil, and seasoning and toss to coat well.

4. Thread shrimp and zucchini onto pre-soaked skewers.
5. Grill the skewers for about 6-8 minutes, flipping occasionally. Serve hot.

Nutrition:
- Net Carbohydrates: 3.2 g
- Protein: 4.1g
- Fat: 9.4g
- Calories: 261

Fried Shrimp Tails

Preparation Time: 10 minutes
Cooking Time: 15 minutes
Servings: 2
Ingredients:
- 1 lb. shrimp tails
- 1 tbsp olive oil
- 1 tsp dried dill
- 1/2 tsp dried parsley
- 2 tbsp coconut flour
- 1/2 cup heavy cream
- 1 tsp chili flakes

Directions:
1. Peel the shrimp tails and sprinkle them with the dried dill and dried parsley.
2. Mix the shrimp tails carefully in the mixing bowl.
3. After this, combine the coconut flour, heavy cream, and chili flakes in a separate bowl and whisk it until you get the smooth batter.
4. Then preheat the air fryer to 330 F.
5. Transfer the shrimp tails to the heavy cream batter and gently stir the seafood.
6. Then spray the air fryer rack and put the shrimp tails there.
7. Cook the shrimp tails for 7 minutes. After this, turn the shrimp tails into another side.
8. Cook the shrimp tails for 7 minutes more. When the seafood is cooked – chill it well. Enjoy!

Nutrition:
- Net Carbohydrates: 2.6 g
- Protein: 5.1g
- Fat: 10.1g
- Calories: 212

Pan-Seared Cod with Tomato Hollandaise

Preparation Time: 10 minutes
Cooking Time: 10 minutes
Servings: 2
Ingredients:
Pan-Seared Cod

- 1 lb. (4-fillets) wild Alaskan Cod
- 1 tbsp. salted butter
- 1 tbsp. olive oil

Tomato Hollandaise

- 3 large egg yolks
- 3 tbsp. warm water
- 226 g salted butter, melted
- 1/4 tsp. salt
- 1/4 tsp. black pepper
- 2 tbsp. tomato paste
- 2 tbsp. fresh lemon juice

Directions:

1. Season both sides of the code fillet without salt, the salt will be added in the last.
2. Heat a skillet over medium heat and coat with olive oil and butter.
3. When the butter heats up, place the cod fillet in the skillet and sear on both sides for 2-3 minutes. Baste the fish fillet with the oil and butter mixture.
4. You will know that the cod is cooked when it easily flakes when poked with a fork.
5. Melt the butter in the microwave.
6. In a double boil, beat egg yolks with warm water until thick and creamy and start forming soft peaks. Remove the double boil from the heat, gradually adding the melted butter and stirring.
7. Season.
8. Mix in the tomato paste. Stir to combine. Pour in the water and lemon juice to lighten the sauce texture.

Nutrition:

- Net Carbohydrates: 3.1 g
- Protein: 18.4g
- Fat: 16.1g
- Calories: 356

Lime Mackerel

Preparation Time: 10 minutes
Cooking Time: 30 minutes
Servings: 2
Ingredients:

- 2 mackerel fillets, boneless
- 2 tbsp. lime juice
- 2 tbsp. olive oil
- A pinch of salt and black pepper
- ½ tsp. sweet paprika

Directions:

1. Arrange the mackerel on a baking sheet lined with parchment paper, add the oil and the other ingredients, rub gently, introduce in the oven at 360 degrees F and bake for 30 minutes.
2. Divide the fish between plates and serve.

Nutrition:

- Net Carbohydrates: 2g
- Protein: 21.1 g
- Fat: 22.7g
- Calories: 297

Turmeric Tilapia

Preparation Time: 10 minutes
Cooking Time: 12 minutes
Servings: 2
Ingredients:

- 4 tilapia fillets, boneless
- 2 tbsp. olive oil
- 1 tsp. turmeric powder
- A pinch of salt and black pepper
- 2 spring onions, chopped
- ¼ tsp. basil, dried
- ¼ tsp. garlic powder
- 1 tbsp. parsley, chopped

Directions:

1. Heat a pan with the oil over medium heat, add the spring onions and cook them for 2 minutes.
2. Add the fish, turmeric, and the other ingredients, cook for 5 minutes on each side, divide between plates and serve.

Nutrition:

- Net Carbohydrates: 1.1g
- Protein: 31.8 g
- Fat: 8.6g
- Calories: 205

Walnut Salmon Mix

Preparation Time: 10 minutes
Cooking Time: 14 minutes
Servings: 2
Ingredients:

- 2 salmon fillets, boneless
- 2 tbsp. avocado oil
- A pinch of salt and black pepper
- 1 tbsp. lime juice
- 2 shallots, chopped
- 2 tbsp. walnuts, chopped
- 2 tbsp. parsley, chopped

Directions:

1. Heat a pan with the oil over medium-high heat, add the shallots, stir and sauté for 2 minutes.
2. Add the fish and the other ingredients, cook for 6 minutes on each side, divide between plates and serve.

Nutrition:

- Net Carbohydrates: 2.7g
- Protein: 35.8 g
- Fat: 14.2g
- Calories: 276

Cioppino

Preparation Time: 15 minutes
Cooking Time: 30 minutes
Servings: 2
Ingredients:

- 2 tbsp. olive oil
- 1/2 onion, chopped
- 2 celery stalks, sliced
- 1 red bell pepper, chopped
- 1 tbsp. minced garlic
- 2 cups fish stock
- 1 (15-oz.) can coconut milk
- 1 cup crushed tomatoes
- 2 tbsp. tomato paste
- 1 tbsp. chopped fresh basil
- 2 tsp. chopped fresh oregano
- 1/2 tsp. of sea salt
- 1/2 tsp. freshly ground black pepper
- 1/4 tsp. red pepper flakes
- 10 oz. salmon, cut into 1-inch pieces
- 1/2 lb. shrimp, peeled and deveined
- 12 clams or mussels, cleaned and debearded but in the shell

Directions:

1. Sauté the vegetables.
2. In a pot, warm the olive oil. Add the onion, celery, red bell pepper, and garlic and sauté until they've softened about 4 minutes.
3. Make the soup base. Stir in the fish stock, coconut milk, crushed tomatoes, tomato paste, basil, oregano, salt, pepper, and red pepper flakes.
4. Boil and then simmer the soup for 10 minutes.

5. Add the seafood. Stir in the salmon and simmer until it goes opaque, about 5 minutes.
6. Add the shrimp and simmer until they're almost cooked through about 3 minutes. Add the mussels.
7. Serve.

Nutrition:
- Net Carbohydrates: 4.2 g
- Protein: 16.4g
- Fat: 11.1g
- Calories: 321

Coconut Mussels

Preparation Time: 10 minutes
Cooking Time: 10-15 minutes
Servings: 2
Ingredients:
- 2 tbsp. coconut oil
- 1/2 sweet onion, chopped
- 2 tsp. minced garlic
- 1 tsp. grated fresh ginger
- 1/2 tsp. turmeric
- 1 cup of coconut milk
- Juice of 1 lime
- 1 1/2 lb. fresh mussels, scrubbed and debearded
- 1 scallion, finely chopped
- 2 tbsp. chopped fresh cilantro
- 1 tbsp. chopped fresh thyme

Directions:
1. Sauté the aromatics.
2. In a pot, warm the coconut oil. Add the onion, garlic, ginger, and turmeric and sauté until they've softened about 3 minutes.
3. Add the liquid. Stir in the coconut milk and lime juice and bring the mixture to a boil.
4. Steam the mussels.
5. Add the mussels to the skillet, cover, and steam until the shells are open, about 10 minutes.
6. Take the skillet off the heat and throw out any unopened mussels.
7. Add the herbs. Stir in the scallion, cilantro, and thyme.
8. Divide the mussels and the sauce between four bowls and serve them immediately.

Nutrition:
- Net Carbohydrates: 1.2 g
- Protein: 1.4g
- Fat: 11.1g
- Calories: 321

Italian Style Halibut Packets

Preparation Time: 10 minutes
Cooking Time: 20 minutes
Servings: 2
Ingredients:

- 2 cups cauliflower florets
- 1 cup roasted red pepper strips
- 1/2 cup sliced sun-dried tomatoes
- 4 (4-oz.) halibut fillets
- 1/4 cup chopped fresh basil
- Juice of 1 lemon
- 1/4 cup good-quality olive oil
- Sea salt for seasoning
- Freshly ground black pepper for seasoning

Directions:

1. Preheat the oven. Set the oven temperature to 400°F.
2. Make the packets.
3. Divide the cauliflower, red pepper strips, and sun-dried tomato between the four pieces of foil, placing the vegetables in the middle of each piece.
4. Top each pile with one halibut fillet, and top each fillet with equal amounts of basil, lemon juice, and olive oil.
5. Fold and crimp the foil to form sealed packets of fish and vegetables and place them on the baking sheet.
6. Bake the packets for about 20 minutes, until the fish flakes with a fork.
7. Be careful of the steam when you open the packet!
8. Transfer the vegetables and halibut to four plates, season with salt and pepper, and serve immediately.

Nutrition:

- Net Carbohydrates: 3.2 g
- Protein: 15.4g
- Fat: 14.1g
- Calories: 313

Greek Tuna Salad

Preparation Time: 10 minutes
Cooking Time: 0 minutes
Servings: 2
Ingredients:

- 3 cans of tuna
- 1/4 small red onion, finely chopped
- 1 celery stalks, finely chopped
- 1/2 avocado, chopped
- 1 tbsp. chopped fresh parsley
- 1 cup Greek yogurt
- 2 tbsp. butter
- 2 tsp. Dijon Mustard
- 1/2 tbsp. vinegar
- Salt and black pepper to taste

Directions:

1. The ingredients listed must be added to a salad bowl and mix until well combined.
2. Serve afterward.

Nutrition:

- Net Carbohydrates: 3.9 g
- Protein: 18.4g
- Fat: 10.4g
- Calories: 376

Blackened Salmon with Avocado Salsa

Preparation Time: 15 minutes
Cooking Time: 10 minutes
Servings: 2
Ingredients:

- 1 tbsp. extra virgin olive oil
- 2 filets of salmon (about 6 oz. each)
- 2 tsp. Cajun seasoning
- 1 med. avocados, diced
- 1 c. cucumber, diced
- 1/4 c. red onion, diced
- 1 tbsp. parsley, chopped
- 1 tbsp. lime juice
- Sea salt & pepper to taste

Directions:

1. The oil must be heated in a skillet.
2. Rub the Cajun seasoning into the fillets, then lay them into the bottom of the skillet once it's hot enough.
3. Cook until a dark crust forms, then flip and repeat.
4. In a medium mixing bowl, combine all the ingredients for the salsa and set aside.
5. Plate the fillets and top with 1/4 of the salsa yielded.
6. Enjoy!

Nutrition:

- Net Carbohydrates: 4.1 g
- Protein: 11.8g
- Fat: 15.8g
- Calories: 425

Tangy Coconut Cod

Preparation Time: 10 minutes
Cooking Time: 10 minutes
Servings: 2
Ingredients:

- 1/3 c. coconut flour
- 1/2 tsp. cayenne pepper
- 1 egg, beaten
- 1 lime
- 1 tsp. crushed red pepper flakes
- 1 tsp. garlic powder
- 12 oz. cod fillets
- Sea salt & pepper to taste

Directions:

1. Let the oven preheat to 400°F/175°C. Then line a baking sheet with non-stick foil.
2. Place the flour in a shallow dish (a plate works fine) and drag the fillets of cod through the beaten egg. Dredge the cod in the coconut flour, then lay it on the baking sheet.
3. Sprinkle top of steak with seasoning and lemon juice.
4. Bake the cod for about 10 to 12 minutes until the fillets are flaky.
5. Serve immediately!

Nutrition:

- Net Carbohydrates: 4.1 g
- Protein: 19.5g
- Fat: 12.1g
- Calories: 318

Fish Taco Bowl

Preparation Time: 10 minutes
Cooking Time: 15 minutes
Servings: 2
Ingredients:

- 2 (5-oz.) tilapia fillets
- 1 tbsp. olive oil
- 4 tsp. Tajin seasoning salt, divided
- 2 cups pre-sliced coleslaw cabbage mix
- 1 tbsp. avocado mayo
- 1 tsp. hot sauce
- 1 avocado, mashed
- Pink Himalayan salt
- Freshly ground black pepper

Directions:

1. Preheat the oven to 425°F. The baking sheet must be lined with a baking mat.
2. Rub the tilapia with olive oil and then coat it with two tsp. of Tajín seasoning salt.
3. Place the fish in the prepared pan.
4. Let the tilapia bake for 15 minutes, or until the fish is opaque when you pierce it with a fork.

5. Meanwhile, in a medium bowl, gently mix to combine the coleslaw and the mayo sauce.
6. You don't want the cabbage super wet, just enough to dress it.
7. Add the mashed avocado and the remaining two tsp. of Tajín seasoning salt to the coleslaw, and season with pink Himalayan salt and pepper.
8. Divide the salad between two bowls.
9. Shred fish into tiny pieces and add to the bowls.
10. Top the fish with a drizzle of mayo sauce and serve.

Nutrition:
- Net Carbohydrates: 2.1 g
- Protein: 17.3g
- Fat: 12.1g
- Calories: 231

Grilled Fish with Zucchini and Pesto

Preparation Time: 10 minutes
Cooking Time: 8 minutes
Servings: 2
Ingredients
For Fish and Zucchini:
- ¾ lb. Whitefish
- 1 Medium-size zucchini, thinly sliced
- 1 tsp Salt
- ½ tsp Ground black pepper
- ½ tbsp Lemon juice
- 1 tbsp Olive oil

For Kale Pesto:
- 1½ oz Kale leaves
- 1 oz Walnuts
- ¼ tsp Minced garlic
- ¼ tsp Salt
- ⅛ tsp Ground black pepper
- 1½ tbsp Lemon juice
- 2/5 cup Olive oil

Directions:
1. Prepare kale pesto and for this, place all the ingredients for the kale pesto in a food processor and pulse for 1 to 2 minutes or until smooth.
2. Tip pesto in a bowl and set aside until required.
3. Place zucchini slices in a bowl, season with ½ tsp. salt and ¼ tsp. black pepper, drizzle with lemon juice and olive oil, and toss until evenly coated, set aside until required.
4. Season fish with remaining salt and black pepper and let sit for 5 minutes.
5. Meanwhile, place a frying pan over medium heat, grease with oil, and let preheat.
6. Pat dry fish with paper towels, brush with oil and add to the frying pan to cook for 3 to 5 minutes per side.
7. When done, serve fish with zucchini and pesto.

Nutrition:
- Net Carbohydrates: 7g
- Protein: 38g
- Fat: 67g
- Calories: 778

Salmon Meatballs

Preparation Time: 10 minutes
Cooking Time: 20 minutes
Servings: 2
Ingredients
The Meatballs:

- 1 lb. salmon skinless and cut into 1-inch pieces
- ½ medium white onion, grated
- 3 tbsp minced cilantro
- 1 tsp minced garlic
- ¾ tsp salt
- ½ tsp ground pepper
- ½ tsp paprika
- ½ tsp ground oregano
- 1 egg white
- ¼ cup and 2 tbsp panko breadcrumbs

The sauce:

- 1 medium avocado, pitted and scooped
- ½ tsp minced garlic
- 2 tbsp minced cilantro
- ¼ tsp salt
- ¼ tsp ground black pepper
- ½ tsp chipotle chili powder
- ½ lime, juiced
- 3 tbsp greek yogurt
- 5 tbsp water

Directions:

1. Set oven to 350°F and let preheat.
2. Meanwhile, prepare meatballs and for this, place salmon in a food processor and pulse for 1 to 2 minutes or until finely chopped.
3. Tip the chopped salmon into a large bowl, add remaining ingredients for meatballs and stir until combined.
4. Shape mixture into four meatballs and then place on a baking sheet greased with oil.
5. Place the baking sheet into the oven and bake for 18 minutes or until nicely golden brown and cooked.
6. In the meantime, prepare the sauce and for this, place all the ingredients for the sauce in a blender and pulse for 1 to 2 minutes or until smooth.
7. Tip the avocado sauce in a bowl and serve.

Nutrition:

- Net Carbohydrates: 7g
- Protein: 35g
- Fat: 12.7g
- Calories: 295

Fried Salmon with Green Beans

Preparation Time: 5 minutes
Cooking Time: 8 minutes
Servings: 2
Ingredients

- 9 oz Green beans, trimmed
- 9 oz Salmon, cut into pieces
- ½ tsp Salt
- ½ tsp Ground black pepper
- 3½ oz Coconut oil

Directions:

1. Place a frying pan over medium heat, add oil and when hot, add beans and cook for 4 minutes.
2. Season beans with salt and black pepper, move them to one side and place salmon on the empty side of the pan.
3. Cook salmon for 3 to 4 minutes per side until nicely golden brown on all sides, stirring beans frequently.
4. When done, slide salmon and beans to a plate, season salmon with salt and black pepper, and serve.

Nutrition:

- Net Carbohydrates: 5g
- Protein: 28g
- Fat: 58g
- Calories: 657

Garlic Butter Salmon

Preparation Time: 10 minutes
Cooking Time: 22 minutes
Servings: 2
Ingredients

- ¾ lb. salmon filet, cut into 4 pieces
- ½ lb. cauliflower florets
- 1 tsp minced garlic
- 1 tsp salt
- ½ tsp ground black pepper
- 1 tbsp chopped parsley
- ½ tsp lemon zest
- 1 tbsp butter, soften
- 1 tbsp butter, melted
- lemon wedges for serving

Directions:

1. Set oven to 400°F, then grease a rimmed baking sheet with butter, place it into the oven and let preheat.
2. Place melted butter in a small bowl, add garlic, lemon zest, and parsley and whisk until combined.
3. Spread cauliflower florets on a heated baking sheet, sprinkle with ½ tsp. salt and ¼ tsp. black pepper and toss until coated.
4. Return baking sheet into the oven and bake for 10 minutes.

5. Then push florets to one side of the baking sheet, place salmon fillet to the other side of the sheet, sprinkle salmon with remaining salt and black pepper on both sides, and then drizzle with the butter garlic mixture.
6. Return baking sheet into the oven and continue baking for 10 to 12 minutes or until fish is cooked through.
7. Serve salmon and cauliflower florets with lemon wedges.

Nutrition:
- Net Carbohydrates: 6.3g
- Protein: 40g
- Fat: 24g
- Calories: 450

Sesame Salmon with Thai Curry Cabbage

Preparation Time: 15 minutes
Cooking Time: 15 minutes
Servings: 2
Ingredients
- 1 Thai curry cabbage
- 15 oz shredded green cabbage
- ½ tsp salt
- ¼ tsp ground black pepper
- ½ tbsp red curry paste
- ½ tbsp sesame oil
- 1 tbsp coconut oil

Lime mayo:
- ¼ lime, juiced and zested
- ½ cup mayonnaise
- 1/8 tsp salt

Salmon:
- 12 oz salmon
- ¾ tsp salt
- ½ tsp ground black pepper
- 1 tbsp sesame seeds
- 1½ oz butter
- ½ lime for serving

Directions:
1. Prepare lime mayonnaise and for this, place all its ingredients in a bowl and whisk until combined, refrigerate sauce until required.
2. Prepare curry cabbage and for this, place a frying pan over high heat, add coconut oil and when hot, add cabbage and stir in curry paste.
3. Cook cabbage for 3 to 5 minutes or until sauté, then season with salt and black pepper, drizzle with sesame oil and remove the pan from heat.
4. Transfer cabbage to a bowl, cover it, and set aside until required, keep cabbage warm.
5. Prepare salmon and for this, cut salmon into pieces, season with salt and black pepper until evenly coated, and then press into sesame seeds.
6. Return frying pan over medium-high heat, add butter and when it melts, add salmon pieces.

7. Baste salmon with melted butter and cook for 3 minutes per side or until cooked.
8. Serve salmon with curry cabbage and lime mayonnaise.

Nutrition:

- Net Carbohydrates: 4.5g
- Protein: 20g
- Fat: 48g
- Calories: 544

Sesame Salmon with Bok Choy

Preparation Time: 1 hour and 10 minutes
Cooking Time: 20 minutes
Servings: 2
Ingredients

- 2, each about 4 oz. salmon fillet
- 1 portobello mushroom cap, ½-inch diced
- 1 small green onion
- 2 baby bok choy, ends trimmed
- ½ tbsp sesame seeds, toasted

Marinade

- ½ tsp grated ginger
- ¼ tsp salt
- ¼ tsp ground black pepper
- ½ tbsp coconut aminos
- ¼ tsp lemon juice
- ½ tbsp olive oil
- ½ tsp sesame oil

Directions:

1. Place all the ingredients for the marinade in a bowl and whisk until combined.
2. Place salmon fillet in a plastic bag, pour in half of the marinade, then seal the bag and turn it upside and down to coat salmon with the marinade and marinate in the refrigerator for 1 hour.
3. When ready to cook, set the oven to 400°F and let preheat.
4. Cut bok choy in half, then place on a baking sheet, add mushrooms, drizzle with remaining marinade and toss until mixed.
5. Add marinated salmon to the baking sheet and bake for 20 minutes or until salmon is cooked through.
6. When done, evenly divide salmon, mushrooms, and bok choy between plates, sprinkle with sesame seeds and serve.

Nutrition:

- Net Carbohydrates: 1.1g
- Protein: 17g
- Fat: 10g
- Calories: 167

Tuna Stuffed Tomatoes

Preparation Time: 10 minutes
Cooking Time: 0 minutes
Servings: 2
Ingredients

- 12 oz. cooked tuna, flaked
- 2 celery ribs, chopped
- ½ tsp. celery salt
- ¼ tsp. ground black pepper
- ½ tsp. dill weed
- ½ cup mayonnaise

Directions:

1. Cut the top of the tomato, about a ¼ inch, and then remove the seeds from inside.
2. Place remaining ingredients, except for sour cream, in a bowl, stir until well mixed and then stuff the mixture into tomatoes.
3. Serve immediately.

Nutrition:

- Net Carbohydrates: 6g
- Protein: 24g
- Fat: 11g
- Calories: 241

Chapter 8: Beef, Pork, and Lamb

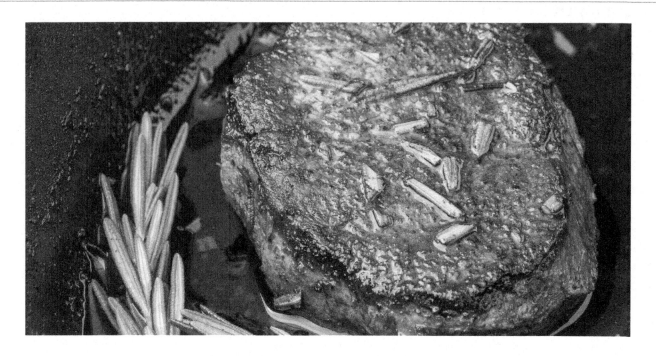

Beef & Cabbage Stew

Preparation Time: 15 minutes
Cooking Time: 2 hours 10 minutes
Servings: 2
Ingredients:

- 2 lb. grass-fed beef stew meat
- 1 1/3 cups hot chicken broth
- 2 yellow onions
- 2 bay leaves
- 1 tsp. Greek seasoning
- Salt
- ground black pepper
- 3 celery stalks
- 1 package cabbage
- 1 can sugar-free tomato sauce
- 1 can sugar-free whole plum tomatoes

Directions:

1. Sear the beef for 4-5 minutes. Stir in the broth, onion, bay leaves, Greek seasoning, salt, and black pepper, and boil. Adjust the heat to low and cook for 1¼ hours.
2. Stir in the celery and cabbage and cook for 30 minutes. Stir in the tomato sauce and chopped plum tomatoes and cook, uncovered for 15-20 minutes. Stir in the salt, discard bay leaves and serve.

Nutrition:

- Net Carbohydrates: 4.9g
- Protein: 36.5g
- Fat: 16g
- Calories: 247

Nut-stuffed Pork Chops

Preparation Time: 20 minutes
Cooking Time: 30 minutes
Servings: 2
Ingredients:

- 3 oz. goat cheese
- 1/2 cup chopped walnuts
- 1/4 cup toasted chopped almonds
- 1 tsp. chopped fresh thyme
- 2 center-cut pork chops, butterflied
- Sea salt
- Freshly ground black pepper
- 2 tbsp. olive oil

Directions:

1. Preheat the oven to 400°F.
2. In a container, stir together the goat cheese, walnuts, almonds, and thyme until well mixed.
3. Season the pork chops inside and outside with salt and pepper.
4. Stuff each chop, pushing the filling to the bottom of the cut section.
5. Secure the stuffing with toothpicks through the meat.
6. Heat oil. Pan sear the pork chops until they're browned on each side, about 10 minutes in total.
7. Put the pork chops into a baking dish and roast the chops in the oven until cooked through about 20 minutes.
8. Serve after removing the toothpicks.

Nutrition:

- Net Carbohydrates: 6.5 g
- Protein: 19.4g
- Fat: 19.5g
- Calories: 425

Roasted Pork Loin with Brown Mustard Sauce

Preparation Time: 10 minutes
Cooking Time: 70 minutes
Servings: 2
Ingredients:

- 1 (2-lb.) boneless pork loin roast
- Sea salt
- Freshly ground black pepper
- 3 tbsp. olive oil
- 1 1/2 cups heavy (whipping) cream
- 3 tbsp. grainy mustard, such as Pommery

Directions:

1. Preheat the oven to 375°F.
2. Season the pork roast all over with sea salt and pepper.
3. Heat oil and then all the sides of the roast must be browned, about 6 minutes in total, and place the roast in a baking dish.

4. When there are approximately 15 minutes of roasting time left, place a small saucepan over medium heat and add the heavy cream and mustard.

5. Stir the sauce until it simmers, then reduce the heat to low. Simmer the sauce until it is vibrant and thick, about 5 minutes. Remove the pan from the heat and set it aside.

Nutrition:
- Net Carbohydrates: 3.1 g
- Protein: 17.4g
- Fat: 18.4g
- Calories: 415

Philly Cheese Steak Wraps

Preparation Time: 10 minutes
Cooking Time: 20 minutes
Servings: 2
Ingredients:
- 2 tbsp. vegetable oil, divided
- 1 large onion, thinly sliced
- 2 large bell peppers, thinly sliced
- 1 tsp. dried oregano
- Kosher salt
- Freshly ground black pepper
- 1 lb. skirt steak, thinly sliced
- 1 cup shredded provolone
- 8 large butterhead lettuce leaves
- 2 tbsp. freshly chopped parsley

Directions:
1. Heat 1 tbsp. oil and put chopped onion and sliced bell peppers and sprinkle with oregano, salt, and pepper.
2. Cook, often stirring, until the onion and pepper are tender, about 3-5 minutes.
3. Transfer the cooked peppers and onions to a plate and add the remaining oil to the skillet.
4. Put the steak in the skillet and spread a single layer, season with salt and pepper.
5. Sear until the steak is seared on one side, about 2-3 minutes.
6. Flip and sear on the second side until cooked through, about 2-3 minutes more for medium.
7. Put the cooked and pepper back to skillet and mix to combine.
8. Sprinkle the cheese over onions and steak.
9. Cover the steak skillet with a lid and cook until the cheese has melted, turn off the heat.
10. Lay the lettuce leaves on a serving platter.
11. Top with steak mixture on each piece of lettuce.
12. Garnish with parsley and serve warm.

Nutrition:
- Net Carbohydrates: 4.3 g
- Protein: 17.5g
- Fat: 15.1g
- Calories: 375

Pork Carnitas

Preparation Time: 5 minutes
Cooking Time: 60 minutes
Servings: 2
Ingredients

- 1-lb. pork shoulder, fat trimmed
- ½ orange, halved
- 1 small jalapeño, deseeded and diced
- ½ medium white onion, peeled and diced
- ¾ tsp minced garlic
- 1 tsp salt
- ¼ tsp ground black pepper
- ½ tsp paprika
- ¼ tsp ground cumin
- ½ tsp dried parsley
- 1 lime, juiced
- 1 tbsp olive oil
- ½ cup of water

Directions:

1. Cut pork into large pieces and season with salt and black pepper.
2. Plugin the instant pot, grease the inner pot with oil, press the 'sauté' button, and when oil is hot, add seasoned pork and cook for 5 minutes per side or until seared.
3. Press the cancel button, add remaining ingredients and toss until mixed.
4. Shut the instant pot with a lid, press the 'meat' button, and cook for 30 minutes at high pressure.
5. When the instant pot beep, do natural pressure release, then open the instant pot and shred pork with two forks.
6. Transfer shredded pork to a rimmed baking sheet, spread evenly, then drizzle with some of the cooking liquid from the inner pot and broil for 5 to 7 minutes or until edges begin to crispy.
7. Serve straight away.

Nutrition:

- Net Carbohydrates: 2g
- Protein: 30g
- Fat: 15g
- Calories: 272

Swedish Meatballs

Preparation Time: 15 minutes
Cooking Time: 20 minutes
Servings: 2
Ingredients:
Swedish Meatballs

- 1-lb. ground beef
- 1 tbsp. dried parsley
- 1/4 tsp. allspice
- 1/4 tsp. nutmeg

- 1/2 tsp. garlic powder
- Salt and pepper to taste
- 1/4 onion, diced
- 2 tbsp. butter

Beef Gravy

- 4 tbsp. butter
- 1 1/2 cups beef stock
- 1/2 cup heavy whipping cream
- 1/2 cup sour cream

- 2 tbsp. Worcestershire sauce
- 1/2 tbsp. Dijon mustard
- Salt and pepper to taste

Directions:

1. Combine the ground beef, dried parsley, allspice, nutmeg, garlic powder, salt, pepper, and onion in a large mixing bowl.
2. Mix the mixture with your hands and shape it into 20 even-sized balls.
3. In a skillet, melt the butter and cook the meatball in batches.
4. Cook the meatball on all sides until golden browned and baste with the butter, set aside.
5. Heat the butter in a pan for the gravy, scrape up the browned bits from the bottom.
6. Add the beef stock, whipping cream, sour cream, Worcestershire sauce, Dijon mustard, salt, and pepper in the pan, then whisk together.
7. Mix the xanthan gum with a ladleful of sauce and
8. Pour in the gravy, stirring continuously.
9. Stir in the meatballs back to the gravy pan, coating the meatballs with the gravy.
10. Simmer for another 15 minutes until cooked through. Serve mashed cauliflower.

Nutrition:

- Net Carbohydrates: 3.1 g
- Protein: 17.5g

- Fat: 10.4g
- Calories: 378

Lamb Chops with Tapenade

Preparation Time: 15 minutes
Cooking Time: 25 minutes
Servings: 2
Ingredients:
For the Tapenade:

- 1 cup pitted Kalamata olive
- 2 tbsp. chopped fresh parsley
- 2 tbsp. extra-virgin olive oil
- 2 tsp. minced garlic
- 2 tsp. freshly squeezed lemon juice

For the Lamb Chops:

- 2 (1-lb.) racks French-cut lamb chops (8 bones each)
- Sea salt
- Freshly ground black pepper
- 1 tbsp. olive oil

Directions:
To Make The Tapenade:

1. Place the olives, parsley, olive oil, garlic, and lemon juice in a food processor and process until the mixture is puréed but still slightly chunky.
2. Transfer the tapenade to a container and store it sealed in the refrigerator until needed.

To Make The Lamb Chops:

1. Preheat the oven to 450°F.
2. Season the lamb racks with pepper and salt
3. Heat oil.
4. Pan sear the lamb racks on all sides until browned, about 5 minutes in total.
5. Arrange the racks upright in the skillet, with the bones interlaced, and roast them for about 20 minutes for medium-rare or until the internal temperature reaches 125°F.

Nutrition:

- Net Carbohydrates: 5.4 g
- Protein: 18.9g
- Fat: 17.4g
- Calories: 387

Sesame Pork with Green Beans

Preparation Time: 5 minutes
Cooking Time: 10 minutes
Servings: 2
Ingredients:

- 2 boneless pork chops
- Pink Himalayan salt
- Freshly ground black pepper
- 2 tbsp. toasted sesame oil, divided
- 2 tbsp. soy sauce
- 1 tsp. Sriracha sauce
- 1 cup fresh green beans

Directions:

1. On a cutting board, pat the pork chops dry with a paper towel. Slice the chops into strips and season with pink Himalayan salt and pepper.
2. In a large skillet over medium heat, heat one tbsp. of sesame oil.
3. Add the pork strips and cook them for 7 minutes, stirring occasionally.
4. In a small bowl, mix the remaining one tbsp. of sesame oil, soy sauce, and Sriracha sauce. Pour into the skillet with the pork.
5. Add the green beans to the skillet, reduce the heat to medium-low, and simmer for 3 to 5 minutes.
6. Divide the pork, green beans, and sauce between two wide, shallow bowls and serve.

Nutrition:

- Net Carbohydrates: 4.1 g
- Protein:18.1 g
- Fat: 15.1g
- Calories: 387

Garlicky Prime Rib Roast

Preparation Time: 15 minutes
Cooking Time: 1 hour 35 minutes
Servings: 2
Ingredients:

- 5 garlic cloves
- 2 tsp. dried thyme
- 2 tbsp. olive oil
- Salt
- ground black pepper
- 1 grass-fed prime rib roast

Directions:

1. Mix the garlic, thyme, oil, salt, and black pepper. Marinate the rib roast with garlic mixture for 1 hour.
2. Warm-up oven to 500 degrees F.
3. Roast for 20 minutes. Lower to 325 degrees F and roast for 65-75 minutes.
4. Remove then chill in 10-15 minutes, slice, and serve.

Nutrition:

- Net Carbohydrates: 0.7g
- Protein: 61.5g
- Fat: 25.9g
- Calories: 499

Beef Taco Bake

Preparation Time: 15 minutes
Cooking Time: 1 hour
Servings: 2
Ingredients:
For Crust:

- 3 organic eggs
- 4 oz. cream cheese
- ½ tsp. taco seasoning
- 1/3 cup heavy cream
- 8 oz. cheddar cheese

For Topping:

- 1-lb. grass-fed ground beef
- 4 oz. green chilies
- ¼ cup sugar-free tomato sauce
- 3 tsp. taco seasoning
- 8 oz. cheddar cheese

Directions:

1. Warm-up oven to 375 degrees F.
2. For the crust: beat the eggs, and cream cheese, taco seasoning, and heavy cream.
3. Place cheddar cheese in the baking dish. Spread cream cheese mixture over cheese.
4. Bake for 25-30 minutes. Remove and then set aside for 5 minutes.

For topping:

1. Cook the beef for 8-10 minutes.
2. Stir in the green chilies, tomato sauce, and taco seasoning and transfer.
3. Place the beef mixture over the crust and sprinkle with cheese. Bake for 18-20 minutes.
4. Remove and then slice and serve.

Nutrition:

- Net Carbohydrates: 4g
- Protein: 38.7g
- Fat: 23g
- Calories: 569

Meatballs Curry

Preparation Time: 15 minutes
Cooking Time: 25 minutes
Servings: 2
Ingredients
For Meatballs:

- 1-lb. lean ground pork
- 2 organic eggs
- 3 tbsp. yellow onion
- ¼ cup fresh parsley leaves
- ¼ tsp. fresh ginger
- 2 garlic cloves
- 1 jalapeño pepper
- 1 tsp. Erythritol
- 1 tbsp. red curry paste
- 3 tbsp. olive oil

For Curry:

- 1 yellow onion
- Salt
- 2 garlic cloves
- ¼ tsp. ginger
- 2 tbsp. red curry paste
- 1 can unsweetened coconut milk
- Ground black pepper
- ¼ cup fresh parsley

Directions:
For meatballs:

1. Mix all the ingredients except oil. Make small-sized balls from the mixture.
2. Cook meatballs for 3-5 minutes. Transfer and put aside.

For curry:

1. Sauté onion and salt for 4-5 minutes. Add the garlic and ginger. Add the curry paste, and sauté for 1-2 minutes. Add coconut milk and meatballs then simmer.
2. Simmer again for 10-12 minutes. Put salt and black pepper. Remove then serve with fresh parsley.

Nutrition:

- Net Carbohydrates: 6.4g
- Protein: 17g
- Fat: 31g
- Calories: 444

BBQ Ribs

Preparation Time: 10 minutes
Cooking Time: 1 hour and 35 minutes
Servings: 2
Ingredients
For Rubs:

- 1/3 tsp onion powder
- 1/3 tsp garlic powder
- 1/3 tbsp salt
- 1/3 tsp ground black pepper
- 1/3 tbsp red chili powder
- 1/3 tbsp paprika
- 1/8 tsp cayenne pepper
- 1/3 tsp dried oregano

Ribs:

- 1/3 rack Pork spare ribs
- 3 tbsp BBQ sauce, unsweetened
- 1/3 cup Water

Directions:

1. Set oven to 425°F and let preheat.
2. Meanwhile, stir all the ingredients for the rub in a bowl until mixed and then sprinkle and rub it generously on all sides of pork ribs until evenly coated.
3. Place seasoned ribs on a roasting pan, pour water in it, and then cover the pan with aluminum foil.
4. Place roasting pan into the oven and bake for 1 hour and 30 minutes or until ribs are tender.
5. Then transfer ribs onto a baking sheet, brush them with BBQ sauce and cook ribs under the broiler for 3 minutes or more until nicely browned.
6. Serve straight away.

Nutrition:

- Net Carbohydrates: 1.3g
- Protein: 33.2g
- Fat: 31g
- Calories: 455

Red Pesto Pork Chops

Preparation Time: 5 minutes
Cooking Time: 15 minutes
Servings: 2
Ingredients

- 2 Pork chops
- ½ tsp Salt
- ½ tsp Ground black pepper
- 1 tbsp Butter
- 3 tbsp Red pesto, divided
- 5 tbsp Mayonnaise

Directions:

1. Brush pork chops with 2 tbsp. red pesto and season with salt and black pepper.
2. Place a frying pan over medium heat, add butter and when it melts, add chops and cook for 9 minutes.
3. Then reduce heat to low heat and simmer pork chops for 5 minutes.
4. Meanwhile, place mayonnaise in a bowl, add remaining pesto and whisk until combined.
5. Serve pork chops with pesto mayonnaise.

Nutrition:

- Net Carbohydrates: 5.4g
- Protein: 37.5g
- Fat: 61g
- Calories: 448

Lamb Chops with Herb Butter

Preparation Time: 5 minute
Cooking Time: 8 minutes
Servings: 2
Ingredients

- 2 lamb chops
- ¾ tsp salt
- ½ tsp ground black pepper
- ½ tbsp butter
- ½ tbsp olive oil

For serving

- 2 oz herb butter
- ½ lemon, cut into wedges

Directions:

1. Place a frying pan over medium heat, add butter and oil, and let heat.
2. Season pork chops with salt and black pepper, add them into the frying pan, and cook for 3 to 4 minutes per side or until nicely golden brown and cooked.
3. Serve pork chops with herb butter and lemon wedges.

Nutrition:

- Net Carbohydrates: 0.3g
- Protein: 43g
- Fat: 62g
- Calories: 729

Cuban Roast Pork

Preparation Time: 10 minutes
Cooking Time: 8 hours and 35 minutes
Servings: 2
Ingredients

- 1½ lb. pork shoulder, boneless and fat trimmed
- ⅓ large red onion, peeled and diced
- 1 tsp minced garlic
- 1 ⅓ tsp salt
- ⅓ tsp ground black pepper
- ⅔ tsp ground cumin
- ⅔ tbsp fresh oregano
- 1 ½ tbsp olive oil
- 1 ¼ tbsp lemon, juiced
- 3 tbsp orange juice

Directions:

1. Place pork shoulder in a shallow dish, season with salt, and set aside.
2. Place remaining ingredients in a food processor, pulse for 1 minute or until smooth, then pour this mixture all over the pork shoulder and massage it into the pork.
3. Cover the dish and marinate the pork in the refrigerator for 8 hours, turning pork halfway through in the marinade.
4. Then remove pork from the refrigerator and let sit at room temperature for 1 hour.
5. Plugin and switch on the slow cooker, place marinated pork in it, fat-side up, then shut with lid, and cook for 8 hours at low heat setting until done.
6. Then transfer pork to a sheet pan and roast it for 30 minutes or until crispy and nicely golden brown.
7. Meanwhile, pour the juices from the slow cooker in a saucepan and cook for 3 to 5 minutes or until the sauce is reduced by half.
8. When pork is ready, shred it with two forms, pour in the sauce, and toss until mixed.
9. Serve straight away.

Nutrition:

- Net Carbohydrates: 6g
- Protein: 59g
- Fat: 70g
- Calories: 912

Garlic Butter Steak

Preparation Time: 10 minutes
Cooking Time: 6 minutes
Servings: 2
Ingredients

- ¾ lb. steak, cut into 4 pieces
- 1 ½ tsp minced garlic
- 1 tsp salt
- ¾ tsp ground black pepper
- 1 tbsp olive oil
- 2 tbsp butter
- ½ tbsp chopped parsley

Directions:

1. Season steaks with salt and black pepper until evenly coated.
2. Place a skillet pan over medium-high heat, add oil and when hot, add seasoned steaks and cook for 3 minutes per side or more until cooked to desired doneness.
3. When done, transfer steaks to a plate and let rest for 5 minutes.
4. Meanwhile, place a skillet pan over low heat, add garlic, season with 1/8 tsp. salt and cook for 4 minutes or until nicely golden.
5. Slice steaks across the grain and evenly divide between two plates.
6. Drizzle steaks with prepared garlic mixture, then sprinkle with parsley and serve.

Nutrition:

- Net Carbohydrates: 1g
- Protein: 37g
- Fat: 31g
- Calories: 429

Chapter 9: Poultry and Eggs

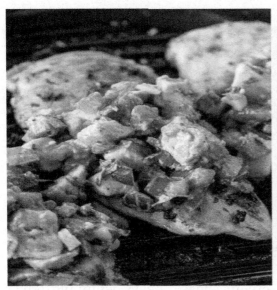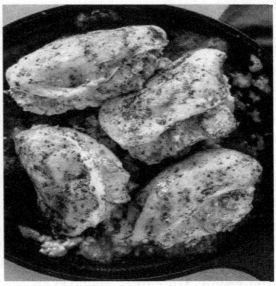

Indian Buttered Chicken

Preparation Time: 15 minutes
Cooking Time: 30 minutes
Servings: 2
Ingredients:

- 3 tbsp. unsalted butter
- 1 medium yellow onion, chopped
- 2 garlic cloves, minced
- 1 tsp. fresh ginger, minced
- 1 1/2 lb. grass-fed chicken breasts, cut into 3/4-inch pieces
- 2 tomatoes, chopped finely
- 1 tbsp. garam masala
- 1 tsp. red chili powder
- 1 tsp. ground cumin
- Salt and ground black pepper, as required
- 1 cup heavy cream
- 2 tbsp. fresh cilantro, chopped

Directions:

1. In a wok, melt butter and sauté the onions for about 5–6 minutes.
2. Now, add in ginger and garlic and sauté for about 1 minute.
3. Add the tomatoes and cook for about 2–3 minutes, crushing with the back of the spoon.
4. Stir in the chicken spices, salt, and black pepper, and cook for about 6–8 minutes or until the desired doneness of the chicken.
5. Put in the cream and cook for about 8–10 more minutes, stirring occasionally.
6. Garnish with fresh cilantro and serve hot.

Nutrition:

- Net Carbohydrates: 6.8 g
- Protein: 12.8 g
- Fat: 14.1g
- Calories: 456

Broccoli and Chicken Casserole

Preparation Time: 15 minutes
Cooking Time: 35 minutes
Servings: 2
Ingredients:

- 2 tbsp. butter
- 1/4 cup cooked bacon, crumbled
- 21/2 cups cheddar cheese, shredded and divided
- 4 oz. cream cheese, softened
- 1/4 cup heavy whipping cream
- 1/2 pack ranch seasoning mix
- 2/3 cup homemade chicken broth
- 11/2 cups small broccoli florets
- 2 cups cooked grass-fed chicken breast, shredded

Directions:

1. Preheat your oven to 350°F.
2. Arrange a rack in the upper portion of the oven.
3. For the chicken mixture: In a large wok, melt the butter over low heat.
4. Add the bacon, 1/2 cup of cheddar cheese, cream cheese, heavy whipping cream, ranch seasoning, and broth, and with a wire whisk, beat until well combined.
5. Cook for about 5 minutes, stirring frequently.
6. Meanwhile, in a microwave-safe dish, place the broccoli and microwave until desired tenderness is achieved.
7. In the wok, add the chicken and broccoli and mix until well combined.
8. Remove from the heat and transfer the mixture into a casserole dish.
9. Top the chicken mixture with the remaining cheddar cheese.
10. Bake for about 25 minutes.
11. Now, set the oven to broiler.
12. Broil the chicken mixture for about 2–3 minutes or until cheese is bubbly.
13. Serve hot.

Nutrition:

- Net Carbohydrates: 4.9 g
- Protein: 14.1g
- Fat: 10.5g
- Calories: 431

Thai Chicken Salad Bowl

Preparation Time: 12 minutes
Cooking Time: 15 minutes
Servings: 2
Ingredients:
Marinade:

- 1 clove garlic, minced
- 1 tbsp. grated ginger
- 1 small red chili, finely chopped
- 1/2 stalk lemongrass, finely chopped
- 2 tbsp. fresh lime juice
- 1 tsp. fish sauce
- 1 tbsp. coconut aminos

Salad:

- 8 oz (226g) (2-pieces) chicken breasts
- 1/2 cup shredded red cabbage
- 1/2 cup shredded green cabbage
- 2/3 cup grated carrot
- 1 tbsp. chopped mint
- 1/2 cup chopped cilantro
- 1 tbsp. chopped chives
- 1/4 cup blanched almonds

Dressing:

- 3 tbsp. extra virgin olive oil
- Salt and pepper to taste

Directions:

1. Oven: 400 F
2. Combine the garlic, ginger, red chili, lemongrass, lime juice, fish sauce, and coconut aminos in a bowl for marinating and crush with a mortar.
3. Flatten the chicken breasts with a meat mallet.
4. Add the chicken to a bowl and add half of the marinade, and coat the chicken evenly.
5. Make it cool in the refrigerator for a maximum of 30 minutes or an hour.
6. Combine both cabbages, carrot, mint, cilantro, and chives in a bowl.
7. In a baking tray, spread out the almonds and roast in the oven for 5-8 minutes, set aside.
8. Grill the chicken in a griddle.
9. Cook through and then slice.
10. Mix in the remaining ingredients.

Nutrition:

- Net Carbohydrates: 3.1 g
- Protein: 12.5g
- Fat: 15.7g
- Calories: 351

Teriyaki Chicken

Preparation Time: 5 minutes
Cooking Time: 18 minutes
Servings: 2
Ingredients:

- 2 chicken thighs, boneless
- 2 tbsp. soy sauce
- 1 tbsp. swerve sweetener
- 1 tbsp. avocado oil

Directions:

1. Take a skillet pan, place it over medium heat, add oil and when hot, add chicken thighs and cook for 5 minutes per side until seared.
2. Then sprinkle sugar over chicken thighs, drizzle with soy sauce and bring the sauce to boil.
3. Switch heat to medium-low level, continue cooking for 3 minutes until chicken is evenly glazed, and then transfer to a plate.
4. Serve chicken with cauliflower rice.

Nutrition:

- Net Carbohydrates: 1 g
- Protein: 17.3 g
- Fat: 9 g
- Calories: 150

Chili Lime Chicken with Coleslaw

Preparation Time: 35 minutes
Cooking Time: 8 minutes
Servings: 2
Ingredients:

- 1 chicken thigh, boneless
- 2 oz. coleslaw
- ¼ tsp minced garlic
- ¾ tbsp. apple cider vinegar
- ½ of a lime, juiced, zested

Seasoning:

- ¼ tsp paprika
- ¼ tsp salt
- 2 tbsp. avocado oil
- 1 tbsp. unsalted butter

Directions:

1. Prepare the marinade and for this, take a medium bowl, add vinegar, oil, garlic, paprika, salt, lime juice, and zest and stir until well mixed.
2. Cut chicken thighs into bite-size pieces, toss until well mixed, and marinate it in the refrigerator for 30 minutes.
3. Then take a skillet pan, place it over medium-high heat, add butter and marinated chicken pieces and cook for 8 minutes until golden brown and thoroughly cooked.
4. Serve chicken with coleslaw.

Nutrition:

- Net Carbohydrates: 1 g
- Protein: 9 g
- Fat: 12.8 g
- Calories: 157.3

Chicken Parmigiana

Preparation Time: 15 minutes
Cooking Time: 25 minutes
Servings: 2
Ingredients:

- 2 (6-oz.) grass-fed skinless, boneless chicken breasts
- 1 large organic egg, beaten
- 1/2 cup superfine blanched almond flour
- 1/4 cup Parmesan cheese, grated
- 1/2 tsp. dried parsley
- 1/2 tsp. paprika
- 1/2 tsp. garlic powder
- Salt and ground black pepper, as required
- 1/4 cup olive oil
- 1 cup sugar-free tomato sauce
- 5 oz. mozzarella cheese, thinly sliced
- 2 tbsp. fresh parsley, chopped

Directions:

1. Preheat your oven to 375°F.
2. Arrange one chicken breast between 2 pieces of parchment paper.
3. With a meat mallet, lb. chicken breast into a 1/2-inch thickness
4. Repeat with the remaining chicken breasts.
5. Add the beaten egg into a shallow dish.
6. Place the almond flour, Parmesan, parsley, spices, salt, and black pepper in another shallow dish, and mix well.
7. Dip chicken breasts into the whipped egg and then coat with the flour mixture.
8. Heat the oil in a deep wok over medium-high heat and fry the chicken breasts for about 3 minutes per side.
9. The chicken breasts must be transferred onto a paper towel-lined plate to drain.
10. At the bottom of a casserole, place about 1/2 cup of tomato sauce and spread evenly.
11. Arrange the chicken breasts over marinara sauce in a single layer.
12. Put sauce on top plus the mozzarella cheese slices.
13. Bake for about 20 minutes or until done completely.
14. Remove from the oven and serve hot with the garnishing of parsley.

Nutrition:

- Net Carbohydrates: 4.1g
- Protein: 15.1g
- Fat: 15.1g
- Calories: 398

Chicken Meatloaf Cups with Pancetta

Preparation Time: 15 minutes
Cooking Time: 30 minutes
Servings: 2
Ingredients:

- 2 tbsp. onion, chopped
- 1 tsp. garlic, minced
- 1-lb. ground chicken
- 2 oz. cooked pancetta, chopped
- 1 egg, beaten
- 1 tsp. mustard
- Salt and black pepper to taste
- 1/2 tsp. crushed red pepper flakes
- 1 tsp. dried basil
- 1/2 tsp. dried oregano
- 4 oz. cheddar cheese, cubed

Directions:

1. In a mixing bowl, mix mustard, onion, ground chicken, egg, bacon, and garlic. Season with oregano, red pepper, black pepper, basil, and salt.
2. Split the mixture into muffin cups—lower one cube of cheddar cheese into each meatloaf cup.
3. Close the top to cover the cheese.
4. Bake in the oven at 345°F for 20 minutes, or until the meatloaf cups become golden brown.

Nutrition:

- Net Carbohydrates: 3.9 g
- Protein: 11.4g
- Fat: 10.4g
- Calories: 231

Bell Pepper Eggs

Preparation Time: 10 minutes
Cooking Time: 4 minutes
Servings: 2
Ingredients:

- 1 green bell pepper
- 2 eggs

Seasoning:

- 1 tsp coconut oil
- ¼ tsp salt
- ¼ tsp ground black pepper

Directions:

1. Prepare pepper rings, and for this, cut out two slices from the pepper, about ¼-inch, and reserve the remaining bell pepper for later use.
2. Take a skillet pan, place it over medium heat, grease it with oil, place pepper rings in it, and then crack an egg into each ring.

3. Season eggs with salt and black pepper, cook for 4 minutes, or until eggs have cooked to the desired level.
4. Transfer eggs to a plate and serve.

Nutrition:

- Net Carbohydrates: 1.7 g
- Protein: 7.2 g
- Fat: 8 g
- Calories: 110.5

Egg Butter

Preparation Time: 5 minutes
Cooking Time: 0 minutes
Servings: 2
Ingredients:

- 2 large eggs, hard-boiled
- 3-oz. unsalted butter
- ½ tsp dried oregano
- ½ tsp dried basil
- 2 leaves of iceberg lettuce

Seasoning:

- ½ tsp of sea salt
- ¼ tsp ground black pepper

Directions:

1. Peel the eggs, then chop them finely and place in a medium bowl.
2. Add remaining ingredients and stir well.
3. Serve egg butter wrapped in a lettuce leaf.

Nutrition:

- Net Carbohydrates: 0.2 g
- Protein: 3 g
- Fat: 16.5 g
- Calories: 159

Eggs in Avocado Cups

Preparation Time: 10 minutes
Cooking Time: 20 minutes
Servings: 2
Ingredients

- 2 ripe avocados, halved and pitted
- 4 organic eggs
- Salt and ground black pepper, as required
- 4 tbsp. cheddar cheese, shredded
- 2 cooked bacon slices, chopped
- 1 tbsp. scallion greens, chopped

Directions

1. Preheat your oven to 400°F.
2. Carefully remove abut about 2 tbsp. of flesh from each avocado half.
3. Place avocado halves into a small baking dish.
4. Carefully, crack an egg in each avocado half and sprinkle with salt and black pepper.
5. Top each egg with cheddar cheese evenly.
6. Bake for about 20 minutes or until the desired doneness of the eggs.
7. Serve immediately with the garnishing of bacon and chives.

Nutrition

- Net Carbohydrates: 2.2 g
- Protein: 13.8 g
- Fat: 16.2 g
- Calories: 343

Garlic Chicken

Preparation Time: 10 minutes
Cooking Time: 40 minutes
Servings: 2
Ingredients

- 1 lb. chicken thighs
- 1 ½ tsp salt
- 1 tsp ground black pepper
- 3½ tsp minced garlic
- ½ lemon, the juice
- ¼ cup chopped fresh parsley
- 2 tbsp butter
- 1 tbsp olive oil

Directions:

1. Set oven to 450°F and let preheat.
2. Meanwhile, take a baking pan, grease it with butter, then add chicken and season with salt and black pepper.
3. Drizzle chicken with lemon juice and oil and sprinkle with garlic and parsley.
4. Place baking pan into the oven and bake for 30 to 40 minutes or until chicken is no longer pink and cooked.

Nutrition:

- Net Carbohydrates: 3g
- Protein: 42g
- Fat: 39g
- Calories: 543

Buffalo Drumsticks

Preparation Time: 15 minutes
Cooking Time: 40 minutes
Servings: 2
Ingredients
For Aioli:

- 5 1⁄3 tbsp mayonnaise
- 1/2 tbsp smoked paprika
- 1/2 tsp minced garlic

For drumsticks:

- 1 lb. chicken drumsticks
- 1/2 tsp salt
- 1/2 tsp paprika powder
- 1/2 tbsp tabasco sauce
- 1/2 tbsp tomato paste
- 1 tbsp white wine vinegar
- 1 tbsp olive oil

Directions:

1. Set oven to 450°F and let preheat.
2. Meanwhile, place drumsticks in a large plastic bag, then whisk together remaining ingredients for drumsticks until smooth and pour over drumsticks.
3. Seal the plastic bag, then turn it upside down until drumsticks are evenly coated with the mixture, and then let marinate for 10 minutes.
4. Then take a large baking dish, grease it with oil and place marinated chicken drumsticks on it.
5. Place baking dish into the oven and bake the chicken for 30 to 40 minutes or until chicken is no longer pink and done.
6. In the meantime, prepared aioli and for this, whisk together all the ingredients for aioli in a bowl until combined.
7. Serve chicken drumsticks with prepared aioli.

Nutrition:

- Net Carbohydrates: 2g
- Protein: 42g
- Fat: 56g
- Calories: 692

Chicken Philly Cheesesteak Casserole

Preparation Time: 5 minutes
Cooking Time: 30 minutes
Servings: 2
Ingredients

- 2⁄3 lb. chicken breasts, 1-inch cubed
- 1⁄3 cup green bell peppers, sliced
- 2 2⁄3 oz mushrooms, sliced
- 1⁄3 cup medium white onions, sliced
- ½ tsp. minced garlic
- 1⁄6 tsp salt
- 1⁄6 tsp ground black pepper
- 2⁄3 tsp Italian seasoning, divided
- 2⁄3 tbsp Worcestershire sauce
- 1⁄3 tbsp butter
- 2⁄3 cup grated cheddar cheese
- 2 2⁄3 oz cream cheese, softened
- 4 oz provolone cheese slices
- 1⁄6 cup mayonnaise

Directions:

1. Set oven to 375°F and let preheat.
2. Meanwhile, take a large skillet pan, place it over medium heat, add butter and when it melts, add chicken and cook for 7 to 10 minutes until chicken golden brown.
3. Meanwhile, place cream cheese in a bowl, add ¼ tsp. garlic, 1/3 tsp. Italian seasoning, Worcestershire sauce, mayonnaise, and cheese and whisk until combined, set aside until required.
4. Add remaining ingredients into the cooked chicken, except for provolone cheese slices, and cook for 3 minutes or until vegetables are tender-crisp.
5. Spoon the chicken mixture into cream cheese mixture and stir until combined.
6. Take a 9 x 13-inch baking dish, add chicken mixture, spread evenly, and then top with cheese slices.
7. Place baking dish into the oven and bake for 15 to 20 minutes or until the top is nicely golden brown, and the mixture is bubbly.
8. Serve straight away.

Nutrition:

- Net Carbohydrates: 5g
- Protein: 26g
- Fat: 40g
- Calories: 489

Butter Chicken

Preparation Time: 5 minutes
Cooking Time: 18 minutes
Servings: 2
Ingredients

- 1/2 lb. chicken breast, 1-inch cubed
- 1/8 medium white onion, peeled and sliced
- 1/4 tsp minced garlic
- 1/2 tsp ginger powder
- 1/2 tsp salt
- 1/2 tsp red chili powder
- 3/4 tsp turmeric powder
- 1/4 tsp ground cinnamon
- 3/4 tbsp tomato paste
- 1 tbsp butter
- 1/2 cup heavy whipping cream

Directions:

1. Place chicken in a bowl, add ginger, salt, red chili powder, turmeric, and cinnamon, and toss until well coated.
2. Place a skillet over medium heat, add butter and when it melts, add onion and garlic and cook for 2 to 3 minutes or until onions are translucent.
3. Increase heat to medium-high level, add the seasoned chicken, and cook for 5 minutes or until chicken is no longer pink and nicely golden brown.
4. Switch heat to a medium low level, then add tomato paste and cream, stir until mixed, and simmer chicken for 5 to 7 minutes or until chicken is cooked fully.
5. Cook chicken curry more for 1 to 2 minutes or until curry is slightly thick.
6. Serve curry with cooked cauliflower rice.

Nutrition:

- Net Carbohydrates: 4.3g
- Protein: 26.5g
- Fat: 26.7g
- Calories: 385

Turkey Soup

Preparation Time: 5 minutes
Cooking Time: 20 minutes
Servings: 2
Ingredients

- 6 oz frozen riced cauliflower
- ½ lb. leftover chopped turkey
- 1 medium celery stalks, diced small
- ½ cup white mushrooms, chopped
- ¼ cup red onion, diced small
- ½ tbsp Italian seasoning
- ¼ tsp onion powder
- ¼ tsp garlic powder
- ½ tsp. sea salt
- ¼ tsp. ground black pepper
- ¼ tsp crushed red pepper flakes
- 1 ½ tbsp chopped parsley
- 1 tbsp olive oil
- 3 cups chicken broth
- ¼ cup heavy cream
- 1 cup shredded Italian blend cheese

Directions:

1. Place a large skillet pan over medium-high heat, add oil and when hot, add onion and celery and cook for 5 minutes or until softened.
2. Add remaining ingredients, except for cauliflower rice, broth, cream, and cheese, stir well and cook for 7 minutes.
3. Pour in broth, simmer the soup for 3 minutes or until heated, then whisk together cream and 1 tbsp. cooking liquid, add it into the pan, and stir well.
4. Simmer the soup for 2 minutes, then add cauliflower rice and ¾ cup cheese, stir until combined, and cook for another 2 minutes or until cauliflower is well heated.
5. Remove pan from heat, ladle soup into the bowl, and top with remaining cheese.
6. Serve straight away.

Nutrition:

- Net Carbohydrates: 4.1g
- Protein: 26.6g
- Fat: 30.4g
- Calories: 409

Chapter 10: Vegetables and Salads

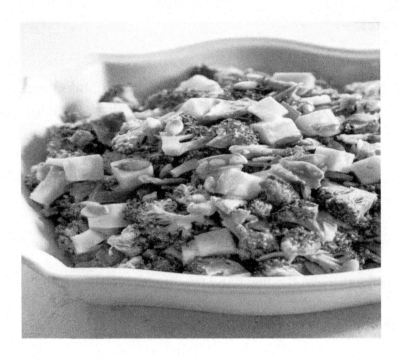

Chili-Lime Tuna Salad

Preparation Time: 10 minutes
Cooking Time: 0 minutes
Servings: 2
Ingredients:

- 1 tbsp. of lime juice
- 1/3 cup of mayonnaise
- 1/4 tsp. of salt
- 1 tsp. of Tajin chili lime seasoning
- 1/8 tsp. of pepper
- 1 medium stalk celery (finely chopped)
- 2 cups of romaine lettuce (chopped roughly)
- 2 tbsp. of red onion (finely chopped)
- optional: chopped green onion, black pepper, lemon juice
- 5 oz canned tuna

Directions:

1. Using a bowl of medium size, mix some of the ingredients such as lime, pepper, and chili-lime
2. Then add tuna and vegetables to the pot and stir. You can serve with cucumber, celery, or a bed of greens

Nutrition:

- Net Carbohydrates: 2.9 g
- Protein: 12.9g
- Fat: 11.3g
- Calories: 259

BLT Salad

Preparation Time: 15 minutes
Cooking Time: 0 minutes
Servings: 2
Ingredients:

- 2 tbsp. melted bacon fat
- 2 tbsp. red wine vinegar
- Freshly ground black pepper
- 4 cups shredded lettuce
- 1 tomato, chopped
- 6 bacon slices, cooked and chopped
- 2 hardboiled eggs, chopped
- 1 tbsp. roasted unsalted sunflower seeds
- 1 tsp. toasted sesame seeds
- 1 cooked chicken breast, sliced (optional)

Directions:

1. In a medium bowl, whisk together the bacon fat and vinegar until emulsified. Season with black pepper.
2. Add the tomato and lettuce to the bowl and toss the vegetables with the dressing.
3. Divide the salad between 4 plates and top each with equal amounts of bacon, egg, sunflower seeds, sesame seeds, and chicken (if using). Serve.

Nutrition:

- Net Carbohydrates: 3.8 g
- Protein: 9.9g
- Fat: 9.4g
- Calories: 287

Wedge Salad

Preparation Time: 10 minutes
Cooking Time: 10 minutes
Servings: 2
Ingredients:

- 4 bacon slices
- ½ head iceberg lettuce halved
- 2 tbsp. blue cheese salad dressing (I use Trader Joe's Chunky Blue Cheese Dressing)
- ¼ cup blue cheese crumbles
- ½ cup halved grape tomatoes

Directions:

1. In a large skillet over medium-high heat, cook the bacon on both sides until crispy, about 8 minutes. Transfer the bacon to a paper towel-lined plate to drain and cool for 5 minutes. Transfer to a cutting board and chop the bacon.
2. Place the lettuce wedges on two plates. Top each with half of the blue cheese dressing, the blue cheese crumbles, the halved grape tomatoes, and the chopped bacon, and serve.

3. If you have a grill, you can drizzle each of your iceberg lettuce wedges with one tbsp. of olive oil, season with pink Himalayan salt and pepper, and grill each side for about 1 minute to add some smoky flavor. Then dress the lettuce wedges as instructed.

Nutrition:
- Net Carbohydrates: 7g
- Protein: 15g
- Fat: 15.5 g
- Calories: 278

Mexican Egg Salad

Preparation Time: 15 minutes
Cooking Time: 10 minutes
Servings: 2
Ingredients:
- 4 large eggs
- ½ cup shredded cheese (I use Mexican blend), divided
- 1 jalapeño
- 1 avocado, halved
- Pink Himalayan salt
- Freshly ground black pepper
- 2 tbsp. chopped fresh cilantro

Directions:
1. Preheat the oven to 350°F.
2. Line a baking sheet with parchment paper or a silicone baking mat.

To Make The Hardboiled Eggs
1. In a medium saucepan, cover the eggs with water. Place over high heat and bring the water to a boil. Once it is boiling, turn off the heat, cover, and leave it on the burner for 10 to 12 minutes.
2. Use a slotted spoon to remove the eggs from the pan and run them under cold water for 1 minute or submerge in an ice bath.
3. Gently tap the shells and peel. (I like to run cold water over my hands as I peel the shells off.)

To Make The Cheese Chips
1. While the eggs are cooking, put 2 (¼-cup) mounds of shredded cheese on the prepared pan and bake for about 7 minutes, or until the edges are brown and the middle has fully melted.
2. Remove the cheese chips from the oven and allow to cool for 5 minutes; they will be floppy when they first come out, but will crisp as they cool.
3. In a medium bowl, chop the hardboiled eggs.
4. Stem, rib, seed, and dice the jalapeño and add it to the eggs.
5. Mash the avocado with a fork—season with pink Himalayan salt and pepper. Add the avocado and cilantro to the eggs and stir to combine.
6. Place the cheese chips on two plates, top with the egg salad, and serve.

Nutrition:
- Net Carbohydrates: 3g
- Protein: 21g
- Fat: 29g
- Calories: 359

Blue Cheese and Bacon Kale Salad

Preparation Time: 10 minutes
Cooking Time: 10 minutes
Servings: 2
Ingredients:

- 4 bacon slices
- 2 cups stemmed and chopped fresh kale
- 1 tbsp. vinaigrette salad dressing (I use Primal Kitchen Greek Vinaigrette)
- Pinch pink Himalayan salt
- Pinch freshly ground black pepper
- ¼ cup pecans
- ¼ cup blue cheese crumbles

Directions:

1. In a medium skillet over medium-high heat, cook the bacon on both sides until crispy, about 8 minutes. Transfer the bacon to a paper towel-lined plate.
2. Meanwhile, in a large bowl, massage the kale with the vinaigrette for 2 minutes. Add the pink Himalayan salt and pepper. Let the kale sit while the bacon cooks, and it will get even softer.
3. Chop the bacon and pecans, and add them to the bowl. Sprinkle in the blue cheese.
4. Toss well to combine, portion onto two plates, and serve.
5. Chopped almonds can replace the chopped pecans.

Nutrition:

- Net Carbohydrates: 7g
- Protein: 16g
- Fat: 29g
- Calories: 353

Chopped Greek Salad

Preparation Time: 10 minutes
Cooking Time: 10 minutes
Servings: 2
Ingredients:

- 2 cups chopped romaine
- ½ cup halved grape tomatoes
- ¼ cup sliced black olives (like Kalamata)
- ¼ cup feta cheese crumbles
- 2 tbsp. vinaigrette salad dressing (I use Primal Kitchen Greek Vinaigrette)
- Pink Himalayan salt
- Freshly ground black pepper
- 1 tbsp. olive oil

Directions:

1. In a large bowl, combine the romaine, tomatoes, olives, feta cheese, and vinaigrette.
2. Season with pink Himalayan salt and pepper, drizzle with olive oil and toss to combine.
3. Divide the salad between two bowls and serve.
4. **Variations:**
5. With Greek salad, there are so many great flavors you can add:

6. Red onion or finely chopped cucumbers for additional crunch and freshness, and chopped pepperoncini for a zesty kick.
7. Finely chopped Genoa salami and pepperoni are good choices.
8. You could replace the feta cheese with goat cheese.

Nutrition:
- Net Carbohydrates: 3g
- Protein: 4g
- Fat: 19g
- Calories: 202

Mediterranean Cucumber Salad

Preparation Time: 10 minutes
Cooking Time: 15 minutes
Servings: 2
Ingredients:
- 1 large cucumber, peeled and finely chopped
- ½ cup halved grape tomatoes
- ¼ cup halved black olives (I used Kalamata)
- ¼ cup crumbled feta cheese
- Pink Himalayan salt
- Freshly ground black pepper
- 2 tbsp. vinaigrette salad dressing (I use Primal Kitchen Greek Vinaigrette)

Directions:
1. In a large bowl, combine the cucumber, tomatoes, olives, and feta cheese—season with pink Himalayan salt and pepper. Add the dressing and toss to combine.
2. Divide the salad between two bowls and serve.
3. This salad can be eaten immediately, of course, but I think it is even better if you cover it with wrap and put it in the fridge to let the dressing marinate the salad ingredients for a few hours.

Nutrition:
- Net Carbohydrates: 4g
- Fat: 13g
- Protein: 4g
- Calories: 152

Avocado Egg Salad Lettuce Cups

Preparation Time: 15 minutes
Cooking Time: 15 minutes
Servings: 2
Ingredients:

- 4 large eggs
- 1 avocado halved
- Pink Himalayan salt
- Freshly ground black pepper
- ½ tsp. freshly squeezed lemon juice
- 4 butter lettuce cups washed and patted dry with paper towels or a clean dish towel
- 2 radishes, thinly sliced

Directions:
To make the hardboiled eggs:

1. In a medium saucepan, cover the eggs with water. Place over high heat and bring the water to a boil. Once it is boiling, turn off the heat, cover, and leave it on the burner for 10 to 12 minutes.
2. Remove the eggs with a slotted spoon and run them under cold water for 1 minute or submerge them in an ice bath.
3. Then gently tap the shells and peel. Run cold water over your hands as you remove the shells.

To make the egg salad:

1. In a medium bowl, chop the hardboiled eggs.
2. Add the avocado to the bowl and mash the flesh with a fork. Season with pink Himalayan salt and pepper, add the lemon juice and stir to combine.
3. Place the four lettuce cups on two plates. Top the lettuce cups with the egg salad and the slices of radish and serve.

Variations:

1. For this recipe, you can incorporate additional ingredients that you may have in your refrigerator or pantry:
2. Add a guacamole vibe to your egg salad with chopped jalapeño and red onion.
3. Chopped bacon adds appealing texture to your egg salad, or add slices of crisp bacon to your lettuce cups.
4. You could also use romaine hearts or baby cos lettuce.

Nutrition:

- Net Carbohydrates: 3g
- Protein: 15g
- Fat: 20g
- Calories: 258

Cabbage Hash Browns

Preparation Time: 10 minutes
Cooking time: 12 minutes
Servings: 2
Ingredients

- 1 ½ cup shredded cabbage
- 2 slices of bacon
- 1/2 tsp garlic powder
- 1 egg

Seasoning:

- 1 tbsp coconut oil
- 1/2 tsp salt
- 1/8 tsp ground black pepper

Directions:

1. Crack the egg in a bowl, add garlic powder, black pepper, and salt, whisk well, then add cabbage, toss until well mixed, and shape the mixture into four patties.
2. Take a large skillet pan, place it over medium heat, add oil, and when hot, add patties in it and cook for 3 minutes per side until golden brown.
3. Transfer hash browns to a plate, then add bacon into the pan and cook for 5 minutes until crispy.
4. Serve hash browns with bacon.

Nutrition:

- Net Carbohydrates: 0.9 g
- Protein: 16 g
- Fat: 29.5 g
- Calories: 336

Cauliflower Hash Browns

Preparation Time: 10 minutes
Cooking Time: 18 minutes
Servings: 2
Ingredients

- 3/4 cup grated cauliflower
- 2 slices of bacon
- 1/2 tsp garlic powder
- 1 large egg white

Seasoning:

- 1 tbsp coconut oil
- 1/2 tsp salt
- 1/8 tsp ground black pepper

Directions:

1. Place grated cauliflower in a heatproof bowl, cover with plastic wrap, poke some holes in it with a fork and then microwave for 3 minutes until tender.
2. Let steamed cauliflower cool for 10 minutes, then wrap in a cheesecloth and squeeze well to drain moisture as much as possible.
3. Crack the egg in a bowl, add garlic powder, black pepper, and salt, whisk well, then add cauliflower and toss until well mixed and sticky mixture comes together.
4. Take a large skillet pan, place it over medium heat, add oil, and when hot, drop cauliflower mixture on it, press lightly to form hash brown patties, and cook for 3 to 4 minutes per side until browned.
5. Transfer hash browns to a plate, then add bacon into the pan and cook for 5 minutes until crispy.
6. Serve hash browns with bacon.

Nutrition:

- Net Carbohydrates: 1.2 g
- Protein: 15.6 g
- Fat: 31 g
- Calories: 347.8

Asparagus, With Bacon and Eggs

Preparation Time: 5 minutes
Cooking Time: 12 minutes
Servings: 2
Ingredients:

- 4 oz asparagus
- 2 slices of bacon, diced
- 1 egg

Seasoning:

- 1/4 tsp salt
- 1/8 tsp ground black pepper

Directions:

1. Take a skillet pan, place it over medium heat, add bacon, and cook for 4 minutes until crispy.
2. Transfer cooked bacon to a plate, then add asparagus into the pan and cook for 5 minutes until tender-crisp.
3. Crack the egg over the cooked asparagus, season with salt and black pepper, then switch heat to medium-low level and cook for 2 minutes until the egg white has set.
4. Chop the cooked bacon slices, sprinkle over the egg and asparagus and serve.

Nutrition:

- Net Carbohydrates: 0.7 g
- Protein: 9 g
- Fat: 15.3 g
- Calories: 179

Omelet-Stuffed Peppers

Preparation Time: 5 minutes
Cooking Time: 20 minutes
Servings: 2
Ingredients:

- 1 large green bell pepper, halved, cored
- 2 eggs
- 2 slices of bacon, chopped, cooked
- 2 tbsp grated parmesan cheese

Seasoning:

- 1/3 tsp salt
- 1/4 tsp ground black pepper

Directions:

1. Turn on the oven, then set it to 400 degrees F, and let preheat.
2. Then take a baking dish, pour in 1 tbsp water, place bell pepper halved in it, cut-side up, and bake for 5 minutes.

3. Meanwhile, crack eggs in a bowl, add chopped bacon and cheese, season with salt and black pepper, and whisk until combined.
4. After 5 minutes of baking time, remove the baking dish from the oven, evenly fill the peppers with egg mixture and continue baking for 15 to 20 minutes until eggs have set.
5. Serve.

Nutrition:
- Net Carbohydrates: 2.8 g
- Protein: 23.5 g
- Fat: 35.2 g
- Calories: 428

Loaded Cauliflower

Preparation Time: 10 minutes
Cooking Time: 8 minutes
Servings: 2
Ingredients
- 1 slice cooked bacon, crumbled
- 1/3 lb. cauliflower florets
- 2/3 tbsp snipped chives
- 1/4 tsp salt
- 1/8 tsp ground black pepper
- 1/8 tsp garlic powder
- 1 tbsp butter
- 1 1/3 oz. sour cream
- 1/3 cup grated cheddar cheese
- 2 tbsp water

Directions:
1. Place cauliflower florets in a heatproof bowl, add water, then cover the bowl with plastic wrap and microwave for 5 to 8 minutes or until florets are tender and cooked.
2. Uncover the bowl, then drain florets and let sit for 2 minutes.
3. Then transfer florets into a food processor and pulse for 1 minute or more until fluffy.
4. Add butter, garlic, and sour cream and blend for 1 minute or more until mashed.
5. Tip mashed cauliflower in a casserole, add half of the cheddar cheese, most of the chives, salt, and black pepper, and stir until combined.
6. Top cauliflower with remaining cheddar cheese, place casserole under the heated broiler, and then cook for 3 minutes or more until the top is nicely golden brown.
7. Top cauliflower with bacon and chives and serve.

Nutrition:
- Net Carbohydrates: 3g
- Protein: 8g
- Fat: 17g
- Calories: 199

Chapter 11: Vegetarian

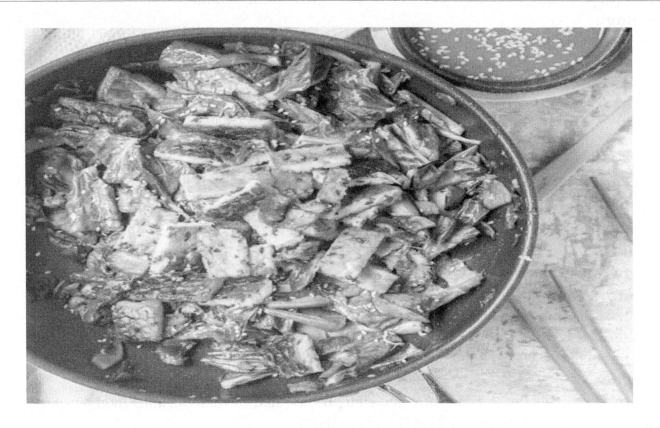

Eggplant Pizza with Tofu

Preparation Time: 15 minutes
Cooking Time: 45 minutes
Servings: 2
Ingredients:

- 2 eggplants, sliced
- 1/3 cup butter, melted
- 2 garlic cloves, minced
- 1 red onion
- 12 oz tofu, chopped
-

- 7 oz tomato sauce
- Salt and black pepper to taste
- 1/2 tsp. cinnamon powder
- 1 cup Parmesan cheese, shredded
- 1/4 cup dried oregano

Directions:

1. Let the oven heat to 400F. Lay the eggplant slices in a baking sheet and brush with some butter. Bake in the oven until lightly browned, about 20 minutes.
2. Heat the remaining butter in a skillet; sauté garlic and onion until fragrant and soft, about 3 minutes.

3. Stir in the tofu and cook for 3 minutes. Add the tomato sauce, salt, and black pepper. Simmer for 10 minutes.
4. Sprinkle with Parmesan cheese and oregano. Bake for 10 minutes.

Nutrition:

- Net Carbohydrates: 4.3 g
- Protein: 10.1g
- Fat: 11.3g
- Calories: 321

Brussel Sprouts with Spiced Halloumi

Preparation Time: 20 minutes
Cooking Time: 30 minutes
Servings: 2
Ingredients:

- 10 oz halloumi cheese, sliced
- 1 tbsp. coconut oil
- 1/2 cup unsweetened coconut, shredded
- 1 tsp. chili powder
- 1/2 tsp. onion powder
- 1/2 lb. Brussels sprouts, shredded
- 4 oz butter
- Salt and black pepper to taste
- Lemon wedges for serving

Directions:

1. In a bowl, mix the shredded coconut, chili powder, salt, coconut oil, and onion powder.
2. Then, toss the halloumi slices in the spice mixture.
3. The grill pan must be heated and then cook the coated halloumi cheese for 2-3 minutes.
4. Transfer to a plate to keep warm.
5. The half butter must be melted in a pan, add, and sauté the Brussels sprouts until slightly caramelized.
6. Then, season with salt and black pepper.
7. Dish the Brussels sprouts into serving plates with the halloumi cheese and lemon wedges.
8. Melt left butter and drizzle over the Brussels sprouts and halloumi cheese. Serve.

Nutrition:

- Net Carbohydrates: 4.1 g
- Protein: 5.4g
- Fat: 9.5g
- Calories: 276

Keto Red Curry

Preparation Time: 20 minutes
Cooking Time: 15-20 minutes
Servings: 2
Ingredients:

- 1 cup broccoli florets
- 1 large handful of fresh spinach
- 4 Tbsp. coconut oil
- 1/4 medium onion
- 1 tsp. garlic, minced
- 1 tsp. fresh ginger, peeled and minced
- 2 tsp. soy sauce
- 1 Tbsp. red curry paste
- 1/2 cup coconut cream

Directions:

1. Add half the coconut oil to a saucepan and heat over medium-high heat.
2. When the oil is hot, put the onion in the pan and sauté for 3-4 minutes, until it is semi-translucent.
3. Sauté garlic, stirring, just until fragrant, about 30 seconds.
4. Lower the heat to medium-low and add broccoli florets. Sauté, stirring for about 1-2 minutes.
5. Now, add the red curry paste. Sauté until the paste is fragrant, then mix everything.
6. Add the spinach on top of the vegetable mixture. When the spinach begins to wilt, add the coconut cream and stir.
7. Add the rest of the coconut oil, the soy sauce, and the minced ginger. Bring to a simmer for 5-10 minutes.
8. Serve hot.

Nutrition:

- Net Carbohydrates: 2.1 g
- Protein: 4.4g
- Fat: 7.1g
- Calories: 265

Sweet-And-Sour Tempeh

Preparation Time: 10 minutes
Cooking Time: 25 minutes
Servings: 2
Ingredients:
Tempeh:

- 1 package of tempeh
- 3/4 cup of vegetable broth

- 2 tbsp. of soy sauce
- 2 tbsp. olive oil

Sauce:

- 1 can of pineapple juice
- 2 tbsp. of brown sugar
- 1/4 cup of white vinegar

- 1 tbsp. of cornstarch
- 1 red bell pepper
- 1 chopped white onion

Directions:

1. Place a skillet on high heat. Pour in the vegetable broth and tempeh in it.
2. Add the soy sauce to the tempeh. Let it cook until it softens. This usually takes 10 minutes.
3. When it is well cooked, remove the tempeh and keep the liquid. We are going to use it for the sauce.
4. Put the tempeh in another skillet placed on medium heat.
5. Sauté it with olive oil and cook until the tempeh is browned. This should take 3 minutes.
6. Place a pot of the reserved liquid from the cooked tempeh on medium heat.
7. Add the pineapple juice, vinegar, brown sugar, and cornstarch. Stir everything together until it's well combined.
8. Let it simmer for 5 minutes.
9. Add the onion and pepper to the sauce.
10. Stir in until the sauce is thick.
11. Reduce the heat, add the cooked tempeh and pineapple juice to the sauce. Leave it to simmer together.
12. Remove from heat and serve with any grain food of your choice.

Nutrition:

- Net Carbohydrates: 2.1 g
- Protein: 5.2g

- Fat: 10g
- Calories: 312

Baked Zucchini Gratin

Preparation Time: 25 minutes
Cooking Time: 30 minutes
Servings: 2
Ingredients:

- 1 large zucchini, cut into 1/4-inch-thick slices
- Pink Himalayan salt
- 1-oz. Brie cheese, rind trimmed off
- 1 tbsp. butter
- Freshly ground black pepper
- 1/3 cup shredded Gruyere cheese
- 1/4 cup crushed pork rinds

Directions:

1. Preheat the oven to 400°F.
2. When the zucchini has been "weeping" for about 30 minutes, in a small saucepan over medium-low heat, heat the Brie and butter, occasionally stirring, until the cheese melts.
3. The mixture is thoroughly combined for about 2 minutes.
4. Arrange the zucchini in an 8-inch baking dish, so the zucchini slices are overlapping a bit.
5. Season with pepper.
6. Pour the Brie mixture over the zucchini, and top with the shredded Gruyere cheese.
7. Sprinkle the crushed pork rinds over the top.
8. Bake for about 25 minutes, until the dish is boiling, and the top is nicely browned, and serve.

Nutrition:

- Net Carbohydrates: 2.2 g
- Protein: 5.1g
- Fat: 11.5g
- Calories: 324

Veggie Greek Moussaka

Preparation Time: 20 minutes
Cooking Time: 30 minutes
Servings: 2
Ingredients:

- 2 large eggplants, cut into strips
- 1 cup diced celery
- 1 cup diced carrots
- 1 small white onion, chopped
- 2 eggs
- 1 tsp. olive oil
- 3 cups grated Parmesan
- 1 cup ricotta cheese
- 3 cloves garlic, minced
- 2 tsp. Italian seasoning blend
- Salt to taste

Sauce:

- 1 1/2 cups heavy cream
- 1/4 cup butter, melted
- 1 cup grated mozzarella cheese
- 2 tsp. Italian seasoning
- 3/4 cup almond flour

Directions:

1. Preheat the oven to 350°F.
2. Lay the eggplant strips, sprinkle with salt, and let sit there to exude liquid. Heat olive oil heat and sauté the onion, celery, garlic, and carrots for 5 minutes.
3. Mix the eggs, 1 cup of Parmesan cheese, ricotta cheese, and salt in a bowl; set aside.
4. Pour the heavy cream into a pot and bring to heat over a medium fire while continually stirring.
5. Stir in the remaining Parmesan cheese and one tsp. of Italian seasoning. Turn the heat off and set it aside.
6. To lay the moussaka, spread a small amount of the sauce at the bottom of the baking dish.
7. Pat dry the eggplant strips and make a single layer on the sauce.
8. A layer of ricotta cheese must be spread on the eggplants, sprinkle some veggies on it, and repeat everything
9. In a small bowl, evenly mix the melted butter, almond flour, and one tsp. of Italian seasoning.
10. Spread the top of the moussaka layers with it, and sprinkle the top with mozzarella cheese.
11. Bake for 25 minutes until the cheese is slightly burned. Slice the moussaka and serve warm.

Nutrition:

- Net Carbohydrates: 3.1 g
- Protein: 5.9g
- Fat: 15.1g
- Calories: 398

Gouda Cauliflower Casserole

Preparation Time: 15 minutes
Cooking Time: 15 minutes
Servings: 2
Ingredients:

- 2 heads cauliflower, cut into florets
- 1/3 cup butter, cubed
- 2 tbsp. melted butter
- 1 white onion, chopped
- Salt and black pepper to taste
- 1/4 almond milk
- 1/2 cup almond flour
- 1 1/2 cups grated gouda cheese

Directions:

1. Preheat the oven to 350°F and put the cauliflower florets in a large microwave-safe bowl.
2. Sprinkle with a bit of water and steam in the microwave for 4 to 5 minutes.
3. Melt the 1/3 cup of butter in a saucepan over medium heat and sauté the onion for 3 minutes.
4. Add the cauliflower, season with salt and black pepper, and mix in almond milk. Simmer for 3 minutes.
5. Mix the remaining melted butter with almond flour.
6. Stir into the cauliflower as well as half of the cheese. Sprinkle the top with the remaining cheese and bake for 10 minutes until the cheese has melted and golden brown.
7. Plate the bake and serve with salad.

Nutrition:

- Net Carbohydrates: 4.1 g
- Protein: 10g
- Fat: 9.4g
- Calories: 349

Spinach and Zucchini Lasagna

Preparation Time: 15 minutes
Cooking Time: 30 minutes
Servings: 2
Ingredients:

- 2 zucchinis, sliced
- Salt and black pepper to taste
- 2 cups ricotta cheese
- 2 cups shredded mozzarella cheese
- 3 cups tomato sauce
- 1 cup baby spinach

Directions:

1. Let the oven heat to 375F and grease a baking dish with cooking spray.
2. Put the zucchini slices in a colander and sprinkle with salt.
3. Let sit and drain liquid for 5 minutes and pat dry with paper towels.
4. Mix the ricotta, mozzarella cheese, salt, and black pepper to evenly combine and spread 1/4 cup of the mixture in the bottom of the baking dish.
5. Layer 1/3 of the zucchini slices on top, spread 1 cup of tomato sauce over, and scatter a 1/3 cup of spinach on top. Repeat process.
6. Grease one end of foil with cooking spray and cover the baking dish with the foil.
7. Let it bake for about 35 minutes. And bake more for 5-10 minutes or until the cheese is a nice golden brown color.
8. Remove the dish, sit for 5 minutes, make slices of the lasagna, and serve warm.

Nutrition:

- Net Carbohydrates: 2.1 g
- Protein: 9.5g
- Fat: 14.1g
- Calories: 376

Cheesy Stuffed Peppers

Preparation Time: 15 minutes
Cooking Time: 40 minutes
Servings: 2
Ingredients:

- 2 tbsp. olive oil
- 4 red bell peppers, halved and seeded
- 1 cup ricotta cheese
- 1/2 cup gorgonzola cheese, crumbled
- 2 cloves garlic, minced
- 1 1/2 cups tomatoes, chopped
- 1 tsp. dried basil
- Salt and black pepper to taste
- 1/2 tsp. oregano

Directions:

1. Let the oven heat up to 350F.
2. In a bowl, mix garlic, tomatoes, gorgonzola, and ricotta cheeses.
3. Stuff the pepper halves and remove them to the baking dish. Season with oregano, salt, cayenne pepper, black pepper, and basil.

Baking Time: 40 minutes
Nutrition:

- Net Carbohydrates: 5.4 g
- Protein: 13.2g
- Fat: 12.4g
- Calories: 295

Stuffed Zucchini Boats

Preparation Time: 15 minutes
Cooking Time: 30 minutes
Servings: 2
Ingredients

- ½ lb. ground beef
- 2 large zucchinis
- ¾ tsp salt, divided
- ¼ tsp ground black pepper
- 1 tbsp Tex-Mex seasoning
- 2 tbsp chopped cilantro
- 1 tbsp olive oil, divided
- 2/3 cup grated mozzarella cheese

Directions:

1. Set oven to 400°F and let preheat.
2. Meanwhile, cut zucchini in half, remove its seeds, then sprinkle with ½ tsp. salt and let zucchini sit for 10 minutes.
3. In the meantime, place a skillet pan over medium heat, add 1 tbsp. oil and when hot, add ground beef to cook for 5 minutes or more until nicely browned.
4. Season beef with salt and Tex-Mex seasoning and cook for 3 minutes or until all the cooking liquid is evaporated.
5. Pat dry zucchini with paper towels, then add cilantro and 1/3 cup of cheese in beef mixture, stir well and then stuff the beef mixture into zucchini halves.
6. Sprinkle remaining cheese on top of stuffed zucchini and place on a baking sheet greased with oil.
7. Place the baking sheet into the oven and bake zucchini for 20 minutes or until the top is nicely browned.
8. Serve straight away.

Nutrition:

- Net Carbohydrates: 3g
- Protein: 16g
- Fat: 25g
- Calories: 300

Creamy Kale Salad

Preparation Time: 15 minutes
Cooking Time: 0 minutes
Servings: 2
Ingredients:

- 1 1/2 tbsp. lemon juice
- 1 cup sour cream
- 1 cup roasted macadamia
- 2 tbsp. sesame seeds oil
- 1 1/2 garlic clove, minced
- 1/2 tsp. black pepper
- 1/4 tsp. salt
- 2 tbsp. lime juice
- 1 bunch kale

Toppings:

- 1 1/2 Avocado, diced
- 1/4 cup Pecans, chopped

Directions:

1. First of all, please confirm you've all the ingredients out there. Chop kale and wash kale, then remove the ribs.
2. Now transfer kale to a large bowl.
3. One thing remains to be done. Add sour cream, lime juice, macadamia, sesame seeds oil, pepper, salt, garlic.
4. Finally, mix thoroughly. Top with your avocado and pecans. Serve& enjoy.

Nutrition:

- Net Carbohydrates: 4.3 g
- Protein: 11.8g
- Fat: 5.1g
- Calories: 291

Chapter 12: Snacks, Sides, and Sauces

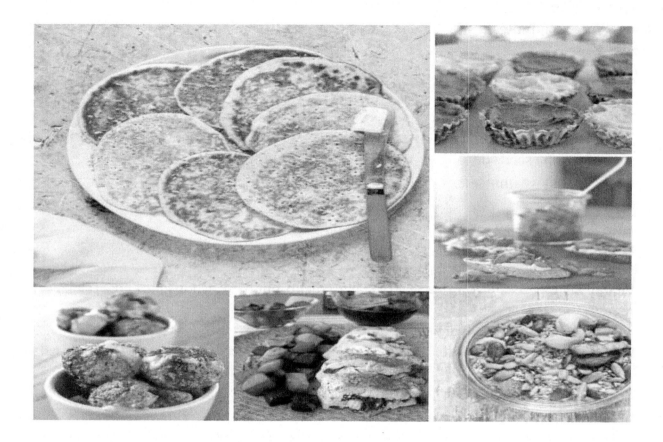

Fried Green Beans Rosemary

Preparation Time: 10 minutes
Cooking Time: 5 minutes
Servings: 2
Ingredients:

- ¾ cup. green beans
- 3 tsp. minced garlic
- 2 tbsps. Rosemary
- ½ tsp. salt
- 1 tbsp. butter

Directions:

1. Warm-up an Air Fryer to 390°F.
2. Put the chopped green beans and then brush with butter. Sprinkle salt, minced garlic, and rosemary over and then cook for 5 minutes. Serve.

Nutrition:

- Net Carbohydrates: 4.5g
- Protein: 0.7g
- Fat: 6.3g
- Calories: 72

Crispy Broccoli Pop Corn

Preparation Time: 15 minutes
Cooking Time: 10 minutes
Servings: 2
Ingredients:

- 2 cup broccoli florets
- 2 cup coconut flour
- 4 egg yolks
- ½ tsp. Salt
- ½ tsp. Pepper
- ¼ cup butter

Directions:

1. Dissolve butter, then let it cool. Break the eggs in it.
2. Put coconut flour in the liquid, then put salt and pepper. Mix.
3. Warm-up an Air Fryer to 400°F.
4. Dip a broccoli floret in the coconut flour mixture, then place it in the Air Fryer.
5. Cook the broccoli florets for 6 minutes. Serve.

Nutrition:

- Net Carbohydrates: 7.8g
- Protein: 5.1g
- Fat: 17.5g
- Calories: 202

Cheesy Cauliflower Croquettes

Preparation Time: 10 minutes
Cooking Time: 16 minutes
Servings: 2
Ingredients:

- 2 cup cauliflower florets
- 2 tsp. garlic
- ½ cup onion
- ¾ tsp. mustard
- ½ tsp. salt
- ½ tsp. pepper
- 2 tbsps. butter
- ¾ c. cheddar cheese

Directions:

1. Microwave the butter. Let it cool.
2. Process the cauliflower florets using a processor. Transfer to a bowl and then put chopped onion and cheese.
3. Put minced garlic, mustard, salt, and pepper, then pour melted butter over. Shape the cauliflower batter into medium balls.
4. Warm-up an Air Fryer to 400°F and cook for 14 minutes. Serve.

Nutrition:

- Net Carbohydrates: 5.1g
- Protein: 6.8g
- Fat: 13g
- Calories: 160

Spinach in Cheese Envelopes

Preparation Time: 15 minutes
Cooking Time: 30 minutes
Servings: 2
Ingredients:

- 3 cup cream cheese
- 1½ cup coconut flour
- 3 egg yolks
- 2 eggs
- ½ cup cheddar cheese
- 2 cup steamed spinach
- ¼ tsp. Salt
- ½ tsp. Pepper
- ¼ cup onion

Directions:

1. Whisk cream cheese, put egg yolks. Stir in coconut flour until becoming a soft dough.
2. Put the dough on a flat surface, then roll until thin. Cut the thin dough into 8 squares.
3. Beat the eggs, then place them in a bowl. Put salt, pepper, and grated cheese.
4. Put chopped spinach and onion in the egg batter.
5. Put spinach filling on a square dough, then fold until becoming an envelope. Glue with water.
6. Warm-up an Air Fryer to 425°F (218°C). Cook for 12 minutes.
7. Remove and serve!

Nutrition:

- Net Carbohydrates: 4.4g
- Protein: 10.4g
- Fat: 34.6g
- Calories: 365

Cheesy Mushroom Slices

Preparation Time: 8-10 minutes
Cooking Time: 15 minutes
Servings: 2
Ingredients:

- 2 cup mushrooms
- 2 eggs
- ¾ cup almond flour
- ½ cup cheddar cheese
- 2 tbsps. Butter
- ½ tsp. Pepper
- ¼ tsp. salt

Directions:

1. Process chopped mushrooms in a food processor, then add eggs, almond flour, and cheddar cheese.
2. Put salt and pepper, then pour melted butter into the food processor. Transfer.
3. Warm-up an Air Fryer to 375°F (191°C).
4. Put the loaf pan on the Air Fryer's rack, then cook for 15 minutes. Slice and serve.

Nutrition:

- Net Carbohydrates: 4.4g
- Protein: 10.4g
- Fat: 34.6g
- Calories: 365

Asparagus Fries

Preparation Time: 10 minutes
Cooking Time: 10 minutes
Servings: 2
Ingredients:

- 10 organic asparagus spears
- 1 tbsp. organic roasted red pepper
- ¼ cup almond flour
- ½ tsp. garlic powder
- ½ tsp. smoked paprika
- 2 tbsp. parsley
- ½ cup parmesan cheese, and full-fat
- 2 organic eggs
- 3 tbsp. mayonnaise, full-fat

Directions:

1. Warm-up oven to 425 degrees F.
2. Process cheese in a food processor, add garlic and parsley and pulse for 1 minute.
3. Add almond flour, pulse for 30 seconds, transfer, and put paprika.
4. Whisk eggs into a shallow dish.
5. Dip asparagus spears into the egg batter, then coat with parmesan mixture and place it on a baking sheet. Bake in the oven for 10 minutes.
6. Put the mayonnaise in a bowl, add red pepper and whisk, then chill. Serve with prepared dip.

Nutrition:

- Net Carbohydrates: 5.5 g
- Protein: 19.1 g
- Fat: 33.4 g
- Calories: 453

Guacamole

Preparation Time: 10 minutes
Cooking Time: 0 minutes
Servings: 2
Ingredients:

- 2 organic avocados pitted
- 1/3 organic red onion
- 1 organic jalapeño
- 1/2 tsp. salt
- 1/2 tsp. ground pepper
- 2 tbsp. tomato salsa
- 1 tbsp. lime juice
- 1/2 organic cilantro

Directions:

1. Slice the avocado flesh horizontally and vertically.
2. Mix in onion, jalapeno, and lime juice in a bowl.
3. Put salt and black pepper, add salsa and mix. Fold in cilantro and serve.

Nutrition:

- Net Carbohydrates: 0.5 g
- Protein: 0.23 g
- Fat: 1.4 g
- Calories: 16.5

Zucchini Noodles

Preparation Time: 5 minutes
Cooking Time: 6 minutes
Servings: 2
Ingredients:

- 2 zucchinis, spiralized into noodles
- 2 tbsp. butter, unsalted
- 1 ½ tbsp. garlic
- 3/4 cup parmesan cheese
- ½ tsp. sea salt
- 1/4 tsp. ground black pepper
- 1/4 tsp. red chili flakes

Directions:

1. Sauté butter and garlic for 1 minute.
2. Put zucchini noodles, cook for 5 minutes, then put salt and black pepper.
3. Transfer then top with cheese and sprinkle with red chili flakes. Serve.

Nutrition:

- Net Carbohydrates: 2.3 g
- Protein: 5 g
- Fat: 26.1 g
- Calories: 298

Cauliflower Soufflé

Preparation Time: 10 minutes
Cooking Time: 12 minutes
Servings: 2
Ingredients:

- 1 cauliflower, florets
- 2 eggs
- 2 tbsp. heavy cream
- 2 oz. cream cheese
- 1/2 cup sour cream
- 1/2 cup asiago cheese
- 1 cup cheddar cheese
- 1/4 cup chives
- 2 tbsp. butter, unsalted
- 6 slices of bacon, sugar-free
- 1 cup of water

Directions:

1. Put eggs, heavy cream, sour cream, cream cheese, and cheeses in a food processor.
2. Put cauliflower florets, pulse for 2 seconds, then add butter and chives and pulse for another 2 seconds.
3. Put water in a pot and insert a trivet stand.
4. Put the cauliflower batter in a greased round casserole dish, then put the dish on the trivet stand.
5. Cook for 12 minutes at high. Remove, top with bacon, and serve.

Nutrition:

- Net Carbohydrates: 5 g
- Protein: 17 g
- Fat: 28 g
- Calories: 342

Simple Marinara Sauce

Preparation Time: 10 minutes
Cooking Time: 1 hour
Servings: 2
Ingredients:

- 1 can 56 oz. crushed tomatoes
- 8 garlic cloves
- 1 tbsp. olive oil
- 2 tsp. salt
- 4 torn basil leaves
- 2 tbsp. balsamic vinegar

Directions:

1. While you could just buy some marinara sauce from the store, the packaged stuff is typically filled with sugar! Now, with some basic ingredients, you will be able to make your own from scratch!
2. You will want to begin by heating a large saucepan over low heat. As it warms up, you can throw in the olive oil, garlic, and basil. Go ahead and sauté until the garlic begins to turn a nice golden color.
3. Next, you will be adding in the tomatoes and gently bring everything to a stew before you add in the salt and reduce the heat.
4. For the next fifty minutes, let the sauce simmer and condense. At the end of this time, you will want to stir in your vinegar, and then your sauce will be set for serving.

Nutrition:

- Net Carbohydrates: 8g
- Protein: 2 g
- Fat: 3 g
- Calories: 80

Green Cilantro Sauce

Preparation Time: 5 minutes
Cooking Time: 20 minutes
Servings: 2
Ingredients:

- 2 cup olive oil
- 1 cup cilantro
- 5 tbsp. water
- 4 garlic cloves
- ¼ tbsp. ground cumin
- Sherry vinegar

Directions:

1. To begin this sauce, you will want to crush your garlic cloves and place them into a food processor along with the cilantro.
2. After you have processed these two ingredients together, slowly begin adding in your olive oil and blend everything together smoothly.
3. If you would like, feel welcome to combine as much or as little water as you would like, along with the sherry vinegar for some extra flavor.
4. Finally, add in your ground cumin, stir, and the sauce will be prepared.

Nutrition:

- Net Carbohydrates: 8g
- Protein: 2 g
- Fat: 3 g
- Calories: 80

Chapter 13: Desserts

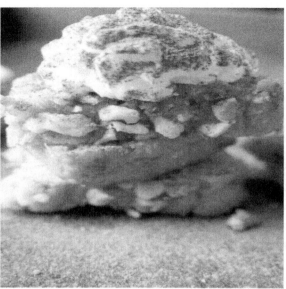 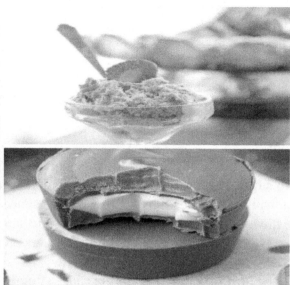

Chocolate Pie

Preparation Time: 15 minutes
Cooking Time: 12 minutes
Servings: 2
Ingredients:

- 2 cups almond flour
- 2 cups heavy cream
- 1/4 cup of cocoa powder
- 3 egg whites
- 3 tbsp. butter, melted
- 3 tsp. Splenda
- 1 tsp. chilled coffee
- 1/8 tsp. liquid Stevia
- Salt

Directions:

1. Preheat the oven to 350 F.
2. Mix the butter with almond flour, ¼ cup cocoa powder, one tsp. of Splenda, Stevia, and a pinch of salt in a mixing bowl, then mix them until they become smooth.
3. Spoon the mix into a baking pan to make the crust and bake it for 12 mins, then set it aside to cool down.
4. Beat the egg whites with 2/3 cup of cocoa powder, two tsp. of Splenda, coffee, heavy cream, and a pinch of salt in a large bowl until they become fluffy and light to make the filling.
5. Pour the filling into the crust, bake it, then chill it in the fridge for 2 hours, then serve it and enjoy it.

Nutrition:

- Net Carbohydrates: 26 g
- Protein: 17.6 g
- Fat: 57.2 g
- Calories: 630

Chocolate Spread with Hazelnuts

Preparation Time: 5 minutes
Cooking Time: 5 minutes
Servings: 2
Ingredients:

- 2 tbsp. cacao powder
- 5 oz. hazelnuts, roasted and without shells
- 1 oz. unsalted butter
- ¼ cup coconut oil

Directions:

1. Whisk all the spread ingredients with a blender for as long as you want. Remember, the longer you blend, the smoother your spread.

Nutrition:

- Net Carbohydrates: 2 g
- Protein: 4 g
- Fat: 28 g
- Calories: 271

Pumpkin Pie Mug Cake

Preparation Time: 5 minutes
Cooking Time: 2 minutes
Servings: 2
Ingredients:

- 2 tbsp coconut flour
- 1 tsp sour cream
- 2 tbsp whipping cream
- 2 eggs
- 1/4 cup pumpkin puree

Others:

- 2 tbsp erythritol sweetener
- 1/3 tsp cinnamon
- 1/4 tsp baking soda

Directions:

1. Take a small bowl, place cream in it, and then beat in sweetener until well combined.
2. Cover the bowl, let it chill in the refrigerator for 30 minutes, then beat in eggs and pumpkin puree and stir in remaining ingredients until incorporated and smooth.
3. Divide the batter between two coffee mugs greased with oil and then microwave for 2 minutes until thoroughly cooked.
4. Serve and enjoy!

Nutrition:

- Net Carbohydrates: 4.6 g
- Protein: 8.8 g
- Fat: 12.1 g
- Calories: 181

Chocolate and Strawberry Crepe

Preparation Time: 5 minutes
Cooking Time: 5 minutes
Servings: 2
Ingredients:

- 1 1/3 tbsp coconut flour
- 1 tsp of cocoa powder
- 1/4 tsp flaxseed
- 1 egg
- 2 ¾ tbsp coconut milk, unsweetened
- 2 tsp avocado oil
- 1/8 tsp baking powder
- 2 oz strawberry, sliced

Directions:

1. Take a medium bowl, place flour in it, and then stir in cocoa powder, baking powder, and flaxseed in it until mixed.
2. Add egg and milk and then whisk until smooth.
3. Take a medium skillet pan, place it over medium heat, add 1 tsp oil and when hot, pour in half of the batter, spread it evenly, and then cook for 1 minute per side until firm.
4. Transfer crepe to a plate, add remaining oil and cook another crepe by using the remaining batter.
5. When done, fill crepes with strawberries, fold them and then serve and enjoy!

Nutrition:

- Net Carbohydrates: 2.8 g
- Protein: 4.4 g
- Fat: 8.5 g
- Calories: 120

Coconut Chia Pudding

Preparation Time: 10 minutes
Cooking Time: 0 minutes
Servings: 2
Ingredients:

- 1/4 cup chia seeds
- 1 1/4 cup coconut milk
- 2 tbsp. unsweetened coconut
- 1 tsp. vanilla extract
- 2 tbsp. maple syrup

Directions:

1. Soak chia seeds in water for 2 to 3 minutes.
2. Take a bowl, add coconut milk, maple syrup, vanilla extract, and chia seeds and whisk them well.
3. Let it aside and mix again after 5 minutes.
4. Put it in an airtight bag and place it in the refrigerator for 1 hour. Serve and enjoy chilled coconut chia pudding.

Nutrition:

- Net Carbohydrates: 1.2 g
- Protein: 3.1g
- Fat: 1.4g
- Calories: 165

Chocolate Mousse

Preparation Time: 15 minutes
Cooking Time: 0 minutes
Servings: 2
Ingredients:

- 8.5 oz. mascarpone cheese
- 2 tbsp. cocoa powder, unsweetened
- 1 tbsp. of a sweetener
- 1 tsp. vanilla extract

Directions:

1. Place mousse in serving cups, serve and enjoy.

Nutrition:

- Net Carbohydrates: 2 g
- Protein: 4 g
- Fat: 27 g
- Calories: 286

Pomegranate Pudding

Preparation Time: 15 minutes
Cooking Time: 10 minutes
Servings: 2
Ingredients:

- 14.5 oz. coconut milk
- ½ cup pomegranate seeds
- 3 tbsp. raw honey
- 2 tbsp. coconut oil
- 1 tbsp. vanilla extract
- 1 packet gelatin, unflavored

Directions:

1. Stir in the honey with coconut milk and vanilla extract.
2. Cook coconut mixture until it starts to boil, then gently add gelatin until completely melted.
3. Stir in the pomegranate seeds and pour the mixture into serving cups, then refrigerate for 4 hours.
4. Serve the coconut pudding and enjoy.

Nutrition:

- Net Carbohydrates: 16.5 g
- Protein: 8.6 g
- Fat: 31.3 g
- Calories: 386

Berry Lemon Cake

Preparation Time: 15 minutes
Cooking Time: 30 minutes
Servings: 2
Ingredients:

- 1/2 cup fresh blueberries
- 1/2 cup coconut flour
- 1/3 cup coconut milk
- 1/3 cup raw honey
- 3 eggs, beaten
- 2 ½ tbsp. coconut oil, melted
- 2 tbsp. fresh lemon juice
- 1 tbsp. lemon zest, grated
- 1 tsp. lemon extract
- 1 tsp. apple cider vinegar
- 1/2 tsp. baking soda
- Salt

Directions:

1. Preheat the oven to 350 F.
2. Mix the apple cider with baking soda in a small bowl.
3. Mix the baking soda mix with coconut oil, lemon juice, and zest, lemon extract, coconut flour and honey, coconut milk, eggs, and a pinch of salt until no lumps are found, then fold in the berries.
4. Pour the batter into a greased baking dish, then bake it for 30 mins.

Nutrition:

- Net Carbohydrates: 12.6 g
- Fat: 13.4 g
- Protein: 3.5 g
- Calories: 203

Keto Frosty

Preparation Time: 45 minutes
Cooking Time: 0 minutes
Servings: 2
Ingredients:

- 1 ½ cups heavy whipping cream
- 2 tbsp. cocoa powder (unsweetened)
- 3 tbsp. Swerve
- 1 tsp. pure vanilla extract
- Salt to taste

Directions:

1. In a bowl, combine all the ingredients.
2. Use a hand mixer and beat until you see stiff peaks forming.
3. Place the mixture in a Ziploc bag.
4. Freeze for 35 minutes.
5. Serve in bowls or dishes.

Nutrition:

- Total Carbohydrate 2.9g
- Protein 1.4g
- Fat 17g
- Calories 164

Keto Shake

Preparation Time: 15 minutes
Cooking Time: 0 minutes
Servings: 2
Ingredients:

- ¾ cup almond milk
- ½ cup ice
- 2 tbsp. almond butter
- 2 tbsp. cocoa powder (unsweetened)
- 2 tbsp. Swerve
- 1 tbsp. chia seeds
- 2 tbsp. hemp seeds
- ½ tbsp. vanilla extract
- Salt to taste

Directions:

1. Blend all the ingredients in a food processor.
2. Chill in the refrigerator before serving.

Nutrition:

- Total Carbohydrate 3.6g
- Protein 1.6g
- Fat 9.5g
- Calories 104

Blueberry Ice Cream

Preparation Time: 15 minutes
Cooking Time: 0 minutes
Servings: 2
Ingredients:

- 1 cup heavy whipping cream
- ½ cup crème Fraiche
- ½ cup blueberries
- 2 egg yolks
- 1 tbsp. vanilla powder

Directions:

1. Whip the whipping cream until it becomes fluffy, then set it aside.
2. Beat the crème Fraiche until it becomes fluffy, then add the whipping cream, vanilla, blueberries, and egg yolks and beat them again until they become creamy.
3. Spoon the ice cream into a loaf pan and freeze it for 1 hour, then serve it and enjoy it.

Nutrition:

- Net Carbohydrates: 3.2 g
- Protein: 2.4 g
- Fat: 19 g
- Calories: 202

Lemon Soufflé

Preparation Time: 15 minutes
Cooking Time: 35 minutes
Servings: 2
Ingredients:

- 2 large organic eggs (whites and yolks separated)
- ¼ cups granulated erythritol, divided
- 1 cup ricotta cheese
- 1 tbsp. fresh lemon juice
- 2 tsp. lemon zest, grated
- 1 tsp. poppy seeds
- 1 tsp. organic vanilla extract

Directions:

1. Preheat your oven to 375°F.
2. Grease 4 ramekins.
3. Add egg whites and beat in a clean glass bowl until it has a foam-like texture.
4. Add 2 tbsp. of erythritol and beat the mixture until it is stiff.
5. In another bowl, add ricotta cheese, egg yolks, and the remaining erythritol until it is mixed thoroughly.
6. Put the lemon juice and lemon zest in the bowl and mix well.
7. Add the poppy seeds and vanilla extract and mix again.
8. Add the whipped egg whites into the ricotta mixture and gently stir.
9. Place the mixture into prepared ramekins evenly.
10. Bake for about 20 minutes.

11. Remove from oven and serve immediately.

Nutrition:

- Net Carbohydrates: 4g
- Protein: 10.4 g
- Fat: 7.7g
- Calories: 130

Lemon Curd

Preparation Time: 10 minutes
Cooking Time: 12 minutes
Servings: 2
Ingredients

- 1/4 cup erythritol sweetener
- 3 1/3 tbsp butter
- 2 lemons, juiced and zested
- 2 eggs, small
- 1 egg yolk

Directions:

1. Take a heatproof bowl, add erythritol, butter, lemon zest, and lemon juice and whisk until just mixed.
2. Place the bowl into the microwave and heat for 30 to 60 seconds or more until butter melts and then whisk well.
3. Whisk in eggs and egg yolks, then place the bowl over a saucepan containing simmering water and continue whisking for 10 minutes until the mixture coats the back of a spoon.
4. Then remove the bowl from the pan and divide evenly between sterilized jars and store them into the refrigerator to chill.
5. Serve when ready.

Nutrition:

- Net Carbohydrates: 2g
- Protein: 7g
- Fat: 25g
- Calories: 258

Chocolate Gelato

Preparation Time: 4 hours
Cooking Time: 15 minutes
Servings: 2
Ingredients

- ½ cup heavy whipping cream
- 3 tbsp erythritol sweetener, powdered
- ¾ tbsp cocoa powder, unsweetened
- 1 egg yolk
- ¼ tsp vanilla extract, unsweetened

Directions:

1. Place a saucepan over medium-high heat, add cream and sweetener, stir until mixed and bring the mixture to boil.
2. Reduce heat to medium-low level, simmer the mixture and then whisk in cocoa powder until well combined, stirring continuously until the mixture starts to thicken.
3. Then remove the pan from heat and cool for 5 minutes.
4. Meanwhile, place the egg yolk in a bowl, add vanilla and whisk until combined, then add into the cooled cream mixture and beat until smooth and frothy.
5. Transfer mixture into a freezer-proof bowl and chill in the freezer for 4 hours or more until set, stirring every hour.
6. Serve when ready.

Nutrition:

- Net Carbohydrates: 4.75g
- Protein: 1.75g
- Fat: 22.5g
- Calories: 231

Chapter 14: Drinks

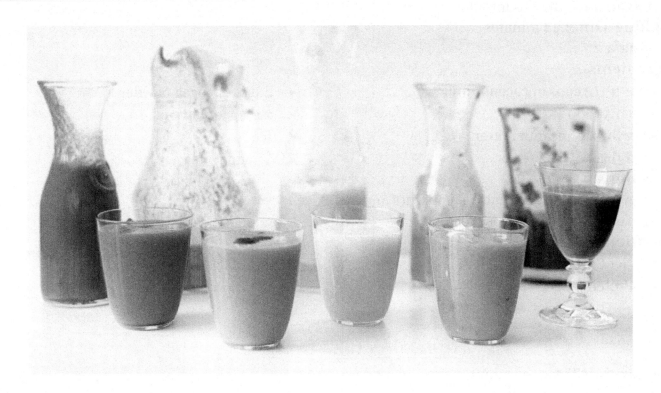

Chocolate Sea Salt Smoothie

Preparation Time: 15 minutes
Cooking Time: 5 minutes
Servings: 2
Ingredients:

- 1 avocado
- 2 cups almond milk
- 1tbsp tahini
- ¼ cup of cocoa powder
- 1 scoop Keto chocolate base

Directions:

1. Combine all the mixture in a high-speed blender. Add ice and serve!

Nutrition:

- Net Carbohydrates: 5,75 g
- Protein: 5.5g
- Fat: 20g
- Calories: 235

Keto Smoothie

Preparation Time: 10 minutes
Cooking Time: 24 minutes
Servings: 2
Ingredients

- 2-2 1/2 cups of coconut milk
- 1 avocado
- 2 tbsp. of peanut butter
- 2 tbsp. of chia seeds
- 4 tsp. of cocoa powder
- 2 tbsp. of olive oil
- Ice
- ½ cup water

Directions:

1. Add all the ingredients in a mixture and blend well.
2. Your keto smoothie is ready.

Nutrition:

- Net Carbohydrates: 3 g
- Protein: 9 g
- Fat: 25 g
- Calories: 237g

Tropical Vanilla Milkshake

Preparation Time: 15 minutes
Cooking Time: 0 minutes
Servings: 2
Ingredients:

- 2 tbsp. of erythritol
- 1 cup of coconut milk
- 1/4 cup of heavy cream
- 1 tsp. of vanilla extract

Directions:

1. Pour in the vanilla extract and erythritol into the blender.
2. Add in the coconut milk, then the heavy cream, and blend for 10 to 20 seconds.
3. Add ice if you'd like or freeze.

Nutrition:

- Net Carbohydrates: 2.9 g
- Protein: 4.2g
- Fat: 9.5g
- Calories: 231

Creamy Cinnamon Smoothie

Preparation Time: 15 minutes
Cooking Time: 0 minutes
Servings: 2
Ingredients:

- 2 cups of coconut milk
- 1 scoop vanilla protein powder
- 5 drops liquid stevia
- 1 tsp. ground cinnamon
- 1/2 tsp. alcohol-free vanilla extract

Directions:

1. Put the coconut milk, protein powder, stevia, cinnamon, and vanilla in a blender and blend until smooth.
2. Pour into two glasses and serve immediately.

Nutrition:

- Net Carbohydrates: 3.7 g
- Protein: 4.1g
- Fat: 3.1g
- Calories: 212

Super Greens Smoothie

Preparation Time: 15 minutes
Cooking Time: 0 minutes
Servings: 2
Ingredients:

- 6 kale leaves, chopped
- 3 stalks celery, chopped
- 1 ripe avocado, skinned, pitted, sliced
- 1 cup of ice cubes
- 2 cups spinach, chopped
- 1 large cucumber, peeled and chopped
- Chia seeds to garnish

Directions:

1. In a blender, add the kale, celery, avocado, and ice cubes, and blend for 45 seconds. Add the spinach and cucumber, and process for another 45 seconds until smooth.
2. Pour the smoothie into glasses, garnish it with chia seeds, and serve the drink immediately.

Nutrition:

- Net Carbohydrates: 3.1 g
- Protein: 8.5g
- Fat: 9.4g
- Calories: 290

Kiwi Coconut Smoothie

Preparation Time: 5 minutes
Cooking Time: 0 minutes
Servings: 2
Ingredients:

- 2 kiwis, pulp scooped
- 1 tbsp. xylitol
- 4 ice cubes
- 2 cups unsweetened coconut milk
- 1 cup of coconut yogurt
- Mint leaves to garnish

Directions:

1. Process the kiwis, xylitol, coconut milk, yogurt, and ice cubes in a blender until smooth, for about 3 minutes.
2. Transfer to serving glasses, garnish with mint leaves, and serve.

Nutrition:

- Net Carbohydrates: 1.2 g
- Protein: 3.2g
- Fat: 1.2g
- Calories: 298

Avocado-Coconut Shake

Preparation Time: 5 minutes
Cooking Time: 0 minutes
Servings: 2
Ingredients:

- 3 cups coconut milk, chilled
- 1 avocado, pitted, peeled, sliced
- 2 tbsp. erythritol
- Coconut cream for topping

Directions:

1. Combine coconut milk, avocado, and erythritol, into the smoothie maker, and blend for 1 minute to smooth. Pour the drink into serving glasses, add some coconut cream on top of them, and garnish with mint leaves. Serve immediately.

Nutrition:

- Net Carbohydrates: 0.4 g
- Protein: 3.1g
- Fat: 6.4g
- Calories: 301

Blueberry Tofu Smoothie

Preparation Time: 15 minutes
Cooking Time: 0 minutes
Servings: 2
Ingredients:

- 6 oz. of silken tofu
- 1 medium banana
- 2/3 cups of soy milk
- 1 cup of frozen or fresh blueberries (divided)
- 1 tbsp. of honey
- 2-3 ice cubes (optional)

Directions:

1. Drain the silken tofu to remove the excess water (silken tofu as a high-water content)
2. Peele and slice the banana. Place the sliced banana on a baking sheet and freeze them. This process usually takes up to 15 minutes. This helps to make the smoothie thicker.
3. Get a blender. Blend the banana, tofu, and soy milk. This usually takes up to 30 seconds.
4. Add 1/2 cup of the blueberries to the banana, tofu, and soymilk. Then blend it until it is very smooth.
5. Put the remaining blueberries. Add honey and ice cubes. Blend it until it is well combined.
6. Serve and enjoy.

Nutrition:

- Net Carbohydrates: 2.7 g
- Protein: 12.1g
- Fat: 9.5g
- Calories: 312

Bulletproof Coffee

Preparation Time: 5 minutes
Cooking Time: 0 minutes
Servings: 2
Ingredients:

- 1 1/2 cups hot coffee
- 2 tbsp. MCT oil powder or Bulletproof Brain Octane Oil
- 2 tbsp. butter or ghee

Directions:

1. Pour the hot coffee into the blender.
2. Add the oil powder and butter, and blend until thoroughly mixed and frothy.
3. Pour into a large mug and enjoy.

Nutrition:

- Net Carbohydrates: 1.2 g
- Protein: 2.3g
- Fat: 9.4g
- Calories: 245

Morning Berry-Green Smoothie

Preparation Time: 15 minutes
Cooking Time: 0 minutes
Servings: 2
Ingredients:

- 1 avocado, pitted and sliced
- 3 cups mixed blueberries and strawberries
- 2 cups unsweetened almond milk
- 6 tbsp. heavy cream
- 2 tsp. erythritol
- 1 cup of ice cubes
- 1/3 cup nuts and seeds mix

Directions:

1. Combine the avocado slices, blueberries, strawberries, almond milk, heavy cream, erythritol, ice cubes, nuts, and seeds in a smoothie maker; blend in high-speed until smooth and uniform.
2. Pour the smoothie into drinking glasses and serve immediately.

Nutrition:

- Net Carbohydrates: 1.4 g
- Protein: 2g
- Fat: 5.1g
- Calories: 290

Dark Chocolate Smoothie

Preparation Time: 10 minutes
Cooking Time: 0 minutes
Servings: 2
Ingredients:

- 8 pecans
- 3/4 cup of coconut milk
- 1/4 cup of water
- 1 1/2 cups watercress
- 2 tsp. vegan protein powder
- 1 tbsp. chia seeds
- 1 tbsp. unsweetened cocoa powder
- 4 fresh dates, pitted

Directions:

1. In a blender, all ingredients must be blended until creamy and uniform. Place into two glasses and chill before serving.

Nutrition:

- Net Carbohydrates: 2.1 g
- Protein: 4.4g
- Fat: 10g
- Calories: 299

Creamy Vanilla Cappuccino

Preparation Time: 5 minutes
Cooking Time: 0 minutes
Servings: 2
Ingredients:

- 2 cups unsweetened vanilla almond milk, chilled
- 1 tsp. swerve sugar
- 1/2 tbsp. powdered coffee
- 1 cup cottage cheese, cold
- 1/2 tsp. vanilla bean paste
- 1/4 tsp. xanthan gum
- Unsweetened chocolate shavings to garnish

Directions:

1. In a blender, combine the almond milk, swerve sugar, cottage cheese, coffee, vanilla bean paste, and xanthan gum, and process on high speed for 1 minute until smooth.
2. Pour into tall shake glasses, sprinkle with chocolate shavings, and serve immediately.

Nutrition:

- Net Carbohydrates: 0.5 g
- Protein: 2g
- Fat: 4.1g
- Calories: 190

Golden Turmeric Latte with Nutmeg

Preparation Time: 5 minutes
Cooking Time: 5 minutes
Servings: 2
Ingredients:

- 2 cups almond milk
- 1/3 tsp. cinnamon powder
- 1/2 cup brewed coffee
- 1/4 tsp. turmeric powder
- 1 tsp. xylitol
- Nutmeg powder to garnish

Directions:

1. Add the almond milk, cinnamon powder, coffee, turmeric, and xylitol to the blender.
2. Blend the ingredients at medium speed for 50 seconds and pour the mixture into a saucepan.
3. Over low heat, set the pan and heat through for 6 minutes, without boiling.
4. Keep swirling the pan to prevent boiling. Turn the heat off, and serve in latte cups, topped with nutmeg powder.

Nutrition:

- Net Carbohydrates: 1.2g
- Protein:1 g
- Fat: 9.1g
- Calories: 254

Keto Avocado Smoothie

Preparation Time: 5 minutes
Cooking Time: 10 minutes
Servings: 2
Ingredients

- 2 cups of coconut milk
- 2 tsp. of vanilla extract
- 1 avocado (without stone)
- 1/2 cup ice
- Stevia

Directions:

1. Mix all the ingredients in a food processor.
2. Blend well.
3. Your keto avocado smoothie is ready.

Nutrition:

- Net Carbohydrates: 1 g
- Protein: 3 g
- Fat: 27 g
- Calories: 230

Keto Blueberry Ginger Smoothie

Preparation Time: 10 minutes
Cooking Time: 5 minutes
Servings: 2
Ingredients

- 12 blueberries
- 1/3 cup coconut yogurt
- 3/4 cup coconut milk
- 2 slices of ginger
- 1 and 1/2 slices of apple
- 1/3 Tbsp. collagen powder
- 3/4 tsp. MCT oil
- Stevia

Directions:

1. In a food processor, add all the ingredients.
2. Blend well until smooth.
3. Your smoothie is ready.

Nutrition:

- Net Carbohydrates: 3 g
- Protein: 12 g
- Fat: 17 g
- Calories: 185

Mint Coco

Preparation Time: 10 minutes
Cooking Time: 5 minutes
Servings: 2
Ingredients

- 8 oz/ 2 cups of coconut milk
- 8 oz/ 2 cups of water
- 1 cup cauliflower
- 1 avocado
- 2 scoops of protein
- 2 tsp. of vanilla extract
- 2 tbsp. of chopped mint
- 2 tbsp. of cocoa powder
- 2 tbsp. of coconut oil
- Dash of cinnamon
- Dash of salt

Directions:

1. In a food processor, mix all the ingredients.
2. Blend well.
3. Your smoothie is ready.

Nutrition:

- Net Carbohydrates: 3 g
- Protein: 12 g
- Fat: 16 g
- Calories: 186

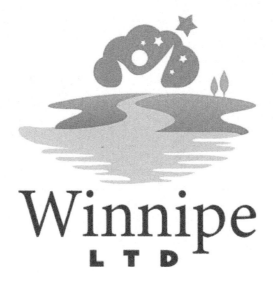

Made in the USA
Monee, IL
18 March 2021

62900070R00072